Mohamed Taieb Frikha
Amine Zouari
Ahmed Tlili

Comparison of adenocarcinoma of the right and left colon

Mohamed Taieb Frikha
Amine Zouari
Ahmed Tlili

Comparison of adenocarcinoma of the right and left colon

Survival and prognostic factors: about 105 cases

Imprint

Any brand names and product names mentioned in this book are subject to trademark, brand or patent protection and are trademarks or registered trademarks of their respective holders. The use of brand names, product names, common names, trade names, product descriptions etc. even without a particular marking in this work is in no way to be construed to mean that such names may be regarded as unrestricted in respect of trademark and brand protection legislation and could thus be used by anyone.

Cover image: www.ingimage.com

This book is a translation from the original published under ISBN 978-620-6-71483-5.

Publisher:
Sciencia Scripts
is a trademark of
Dodo Books Indian Ocean Ltd. and OmniScriptum S.R.L publishing group

120 High Road, East Finchley, London, N2 9ED, United Kingdom
Str. Armeneasca 28/1, office 1, Chisinau MD-2012, Republic of Moldova, Europe
Printed at: see last page
ISBN: 978-620-7-75024-5

Plan

"

INTRODUCTION

According to the World Health Organization, colorectal cancer is the 3rd most common cancer worldwide, with 1.93 million new cases in 2020, and the 2nd leading cause of cancer deaths, with 935,000 deaths in 2020.(1). In Tunisia, colon cancer represents a public health problem due to its ever-increasing frequency. According to data from the Northern Cancer Registry 2007-2009, the trend in colon cancer was upward between 1994 and 2009 in both sexes, with an average annual percentage change equal to 4.5% for both sexes.(2).

The distinction between colon and rectal cancer is well established, with a better prognosis in favor of colon cancer (3). However, the distinction between right and left colon cancer remains controversial. For many years, colon cancer was regarded as a single disease, irrespective of location. Over the past decade, the literature has suggested a difference in prognosis between right and left colon cancer. This has been explained by various factors, notably genetic, environmental and embryological. As a result, they have challenged the notion of the "colon cancer" entity and considered it a highly heterogeneous neoplastic disease(4).

Indeed, a better understanding of the clinico-pathological elements and the distinction of prognostic factors for each site of colon cancer (right and left) could refine therapeutic management, thereby improving prognosis.

With this in mind, we conducted this study to assess the epidemiological, clinical, histological and prognostic profile of adenocarcinomas of the right and left colon, in order to identify the characteristics of each location and its impact on survival.

The main objective of our study is to investigate the impact of right or left location of primary colon adenocarcinoma on patient prognosis (overall survival and recurrence-free survival) after curative surgery.

The secondary objective is to assess the epidemiological, clinical and histological profile of each tumor site.

MATERIALS AND METHODS

---

1. TYPE OF STUDY

This is a mono-centric descriptive and comparative retrospective study from January 1er 2013 to December 31 2017, i.e. a duration of 5 years, involving patients operated on for colon cancer, in the general surgery department of the Habib Bourguiba University Hospital in Sfax.

1.1. Inclusion criteria

We included all patients who had undergone emergency or cold surgery for colonic adenocarcinoma with histological confirmation by pathological examination of the surgical specimen.

1.2. Non-inclusion criteria

We did not include patients with the following criteria in our study:

- Colonic tumors other than adenocarcinomas.
- Patients with recurrent colorectal cancer.
- Tumors of the ileo-caecal valve defined by intraoperative findings.
- Recto-sigmoid hinge tumors defined as tumors located 15 cm from the anal margin on preoperative rectoscopy and/or at the level of the third sacral vertebra on CT and/or, according to intraoperative findings, at the level of the disappearing colonic bands.
- The presence of a double synchronous tumor localization on the right and left.
- Patients with unresectable tumors with locoregional invasion preventing monobloc resection, or with ascites with positive tumor cytology.
- Non-operable patients.
- Hereditary forms: LYNCH and PAF.
- Colonic cancers associated with chronic inflammatory bowel disease (UC and Crohn's).

1.3. Exclusion criteria

- All files where major data were missing, rendering them unusable.
- Patients with a colon tumor that meets the inclusion criteria and who have not undergone surgery.
- Patients lost to follow-up.

2. STUDY APPROACH

2.1. Data collection

Data collection was based on the study of surgical records and reports. The data from each observation were recorded on an anonymous numbered form containing a set of variables. We consulted the files of the carcinology department of the Habib Bourguiba University Hospital in Sfax to collect data on adjuvant treatment and long-term follow-up. All information was recorded, collated and analyzed.

2.2. Study variables

2.2.1. Variable definition

Tumour location: The various studies published on the laterality of colon cancer have defined the colonic anatomical division in two ways. Some authors have considered transverse colonic localization as a straight localization (5) (6) . Others have considered tumours in the proximal 2/3 of the transverse colon to be right-sided, and those in the distal 1/3 of the transverse colon to be left-sided. (7) (8). The latter choice seems more logical, as this subdivision was chosen because of the embryological basis of colonic division and, above all, because of the arterial vascularization of each colonic portion. Indeed, the right colon, including the proximal 2/3 of the transverse, is vascularized by colonic branches originating from the right edge of the superior mesenteric artery, whereas the left colon, including the distal 1/3 of the transverse, is vascularized by the inferior mesenteric artery. (9).

We have chosen the localization of colonic adenocarcinoma based on intraoperative data.

> o Right colon cancer (RCC): cancer that develops in the coecum, ascending colon, right colonic angle and the proximal 2/3 of the transverse colon.
> o Left colon cancer (LCC): cancer that develops in the distal 1/3 of the transverse colon, the left colonic angle, the descending colon and the sigmoid.

- Unresectable tumor: locally advanced tumor based on preoperative workup or intraoperative findings, preventing monobloc resection.
- Altered general condition (AEG): the presence of asthenia and/or anorexia and/or weight loss.
- Anemia: According to the WHO, anemia is defined as a hemoglobin level of less than 13g/dl in men and less than 12g/dl in women. In our study, and with reference to the literature, we defined anemia as a hemoglobin level below 10g/dl, which has been identified as the limiting value conditioning prognosis (10-12)
- Hypo albuminemia: an albumin level below 35mg/l.
- Large tumor: the definition of a large tumor is highly heterogeneous in the literature. Some suggest that a large tumor is defined by a size greater than 3 cm, while others define it as 4 to 5 cm. We therefore studied this parameter in terms of 3 classes: >3cm, >4cm and >5cm.
- Resectable liver metastasis: Class I liver metastasis resectable at the expense of wedge lumpectomy or non-major hepatectomy (involving 1 or 2 segments).

- Overall morbidity: occurrence of one or more postoperative complications (medical, non-specific surgical and specific surgical) within 30 days of surgery.
- Post-operative mortality: death within 30 days of surgery.
- Overall survival (OS): Percentage of patients alive at 3 and 5 years after curative surgery. This is the most common way of expressing, studying and comparing survival.
- Recurrence-free survival (RFS) (disease-free survival (DFS)): Percentage of patients alive and disease-free at 3 and 5 years. Disease-free survival was defined by the presence of a new tumor lesion at the local or distant site after treatment considered curative.

2.2.2. Preoperative variables

- Age
- Gender
- Lifestyle habits (obesity, smoking, alcohol, excessive meat consumption)
- Past history (hypertension, diabetes, heart disease, lung disease, chronic renal failure)
- ASA score (American Society of Anesthesiologists) (Appendix 1)
- Circumstances of discovery (endoscopic surveillance, screening, incidental, clinical symptoms)
- Clinical symptoms (hemorrhage, diarrhea, constipation, pain, weight loss, occlusion, peritonitis) and physical examination (altered general condition, abdominal mass, ascites, jaundice, rectal examination)
- Biological data (hemoglobin, albuminemia, carcinoembryonic antigen (CEA)) and para-clinical data (colonoscopy, thoracoabdominopelvic computed tomography (TAP CT), chest x-

ray, abdominal ultrasound, hepatic magnetic resonance imaging
(MRI)).

- Near upstream stoma.

2.2.3. Operating variables

- Transfusion
- Circumstances of surgery (cold, emergency)
    - o If emergency :   (occlusion,   septic   complication,
      bleeding)
- Surgical approach (laparoscopic or open)
- Intraoperative investigation (carcinosis, adenopathies, metastases,
  ascites, locoregional invasion, perforated tumor, occlusion)
- Tumor location and size
- Surgical procedure (right colectomy, left colectomy, high or low
  segmental colectomy, total colectomy)
- Operating time

2.2.4. Post-operative variables

- Postoperative length of stay;
- Post-operative death
- Post-operative care (simple or complicated)
- Pathological examination of the surgical specimen (TNM stage
  (Appendix 2), quality of resection, number of lymph nodes
  removed, presence of peri-nervous sheathing, presence of vascular
  emboli, immunohistochemistry and molecular biology studies).
- Chemotherapy (type, protocol)
- Long-term outcome (locoregional or distant recurrence, death)
- Follow-up time

2.3. Data processing and statistical analysis

All data were entered using SPSS software (Statistical Package for the Social Science Version 20). We carried out a descriptive study followed by an analytical study.

2.3.1. Descriptive analysis

Quantitative variables were expressed by the mean when the distribution was Gaussian, and by the median and extreme values when the distribution did not follow the normal distribution.

Categorical variables were described by calculating observed numbers and relative frequencies (percentages).

2.3.2. Comparative analysis

We conducted a comparative study comparing the right colon adenocarcinoma group with the left colon adenocarcinoma group.

The Pearson chi-square test was used to study the relationship (p) between two categorical variables. If the conditions, notably sample normality, were not applicable, Fisher's exact test was used.

Student's parametric test was applied to compare means when the distribution is normal with equal variance. The non-parametric Mann Whitney test was applied to compare two means when the conditions for using the first test were not met.

The significance threshold was set at 95% ($p < 0.050$) for the various tests performed.

Survival was studied using the Kaplan Meier method, with median survival compared using the Log-Rank test ($p < 0.05$).

2.4. Bibliographic research

A bibliographic search was carried out in electronic databases (PubMed, Science direct and Google Scholar) with the key words: adenocarcinoma, colon cancer, right colon, left colon, survival, prognostic factors in French and English up to May 2022.

RESULTS

1. DESCRIPTIVE STUDY

1.1. EPIDEMIOLOGICAL CHARACTERISTICS OF THE POPULATION

1.1.1. Patient distribution by tumor location

Our sample included 105 people, of whom 27 (26%) had right-colon tumors and 78 (74%) had left-colon tumors.

1.1.2. Patient distribution by age and gender

The age range of the patients studied was 40 to 86 years, divided into 52 men (49.5%) and 53 women (50.5%).

The following table (Table I) illustrates the age and gender distribution for both right and left colon cancer groups:

Table IPatient distribution by age and gender

Variable	Right colon	Left colon	Total
Gender **n (%)**			
Men	16 (59%)	36 (46%)	52 (49.5%)
Women	11 (41%)	42 (54%)	53 (50,47%)
Ratio	**1.45**	**0.85**	**0.98**
Age Average (years) [Min-Max]	67 [49-84]	64 [40-86]	64,7 [40-86]

1.1.3. Distribution of patients by history and habits

The study of risk factors showed the presence of a family history of colorectal cancer in 6 patients and the presence of a personal history of polyps in 9 patients. The study of exogenous risk factors showed that 30%

of patients were obese, and 42.8% were smokers. The distribution according to location is detailed in Table II.

Table IIDistribution of patients according to risk factors

History	Right colon	Left colon	Total
Family history* of colorectal cancer	2	4	6
Polyps	1	8	9
Resection	1	5	6
No resection	0	3	3
Obesity (n(%))			
Yes	5 (18,5%)	25 (32%)	30 (28,5%)
No	10 (37%)	24 (30,7%)	34 (32,4%)
Tobacco (n(%))			
Yes	15(55,5%)	30 (38,4%)	45(42,8%)
No	12 (44,4%)	48(61,5%)	60(57,1%)
Alcohol (n(%))			
Yes	4 (14,8%)	13 (16,6%)	17 (16,2%)
No	23 (85,1%)	65 (83,3%)	88 (83,8%)

*antecedent

o Terrain and comorbidities:

The ASA score is divided in our population into: 49 (46.6%) patients ASA I, 49 (46.6%) patients also ASA II and the remainder (7 patients: 6.6%) have an ASA III score (figure 1).

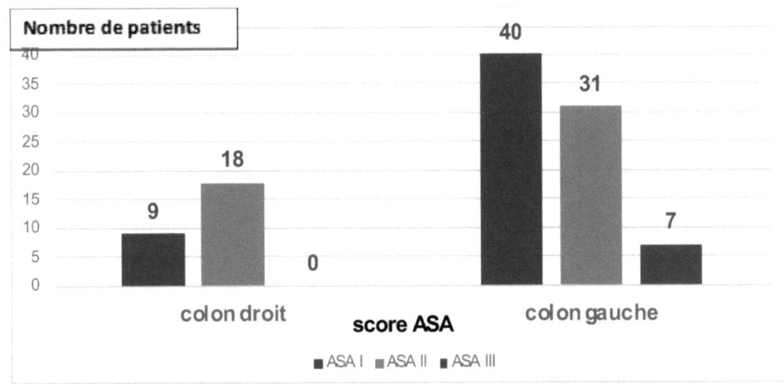

Figure 1ASA score distribution by tumor location

The study of comorbidities showed that 33 patients were hypertensive, 21 patients were diabetic, 8 patients had heart disease, 2 patients had lung disease and 1 patient had chronic renal failure. The distribution according to location is detailed in Figure 2.

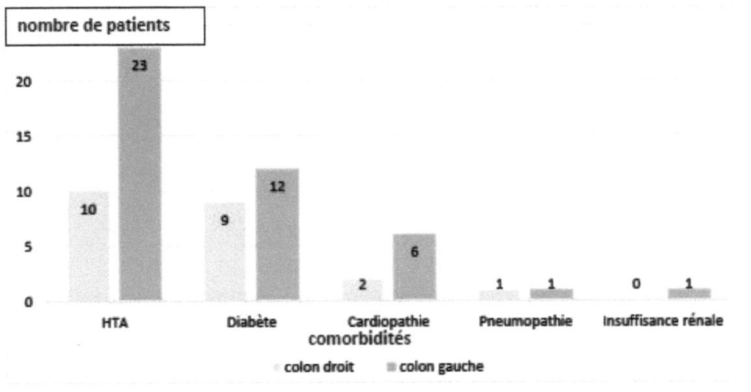

Figure 2Comorbidities by tumor site

1.2. CLINICAL AND PARACLINICAL CHARACTERISTICS

1.2.1. Circumstances of discovery

Endoscopic surveillance after endoscopic polypectomy was noted as the circumstance of discovery in 4 (3%) patients. The other circumstances of discovery were clinical symptoms (Table III).

Table IIIDistribution of circumstances of discovery according to tumour location

Functional sign (n (%))	Right colon	Left colon	Total
Abdominal pain	23 (85,2%)	60 (76,9%)	83 (79%)
Transit disorders	18 (66,6%)	49 (62,8%)	67 (63,8%)
AEG*	16 (59,2%)	42 (53,8%)	58 (55,2%)
Lower digestive hemorrhage (LHD)**	3 (11,1%)	13 (16,6%)	16 (15,2%)
A revealing complication	*13 (48,1%)*	38 (48,7%)	51 (48,5%)

* AEG: Impaired general condition
** low abundance

The tumor was discovered by a complication in 51 patients (48.5%) (Figure 3). It should be noted that our series did not include any patients presenting a complication such as moderate and/or severe digestive haemorrhage requiring medical treatment and/or emergency surgery.

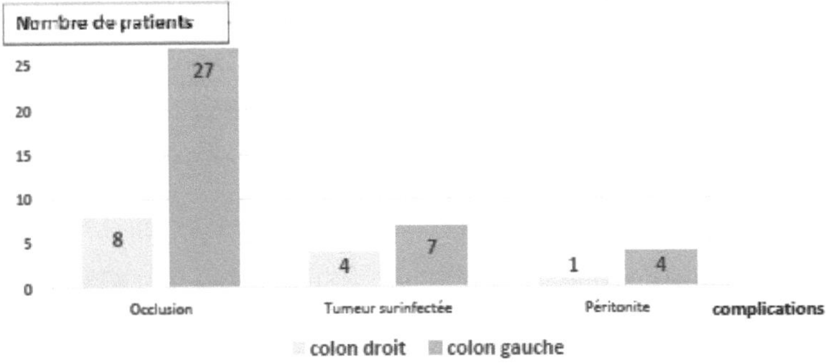

Figure 3Complicated forms according to tumor location

1.2.2. Endoscopic and radiological characteristics

1.2.2.1. Lower GI endoscopy

All cold surgery patients (54 patients (51.4%)) underwent colonoscopy. Colonoscopy was total in 92.3% of patients with right-sided colon cancer and in 62.8% of patients with left-sided colon cancer. Colonoscopy was not total in 17 cases because of a stenosing tumor. Three patients underwent colonoscopy after near-upper colostomy. It was complete by exploring the colon proximal to the tumor through the colostomy orifice and the distal part through the anus. The tumour was ulcerating in 67.8% of cases (Table IV).

Table IVDistribution of endoscopic findings by tumor location

Exploration (n(%))	Right colon	Left colon	Total
Colonoscopy	13 (48,1%)	43 (55,1%)	56 (53,3%)
Total	12 (92,3%)	27 (62,8%)	39 (69,6%)
Tumor appearance	12 (92,3%)	26 (60,4%)	38 (67,8%)
Ulcerative budding	1 (7,7%)	17 (39,5%)	18 (32,1%)
Stenosing			

1.2.2.2.   Thoracic-Abdomino-Pelvic scanner

CAT scans were performed in 100% of patients. It showed tumour extension to neighbouring organs in 8 cases and liver metastases in 17 patients. The distribution according to laterality is detailed in Table V.

Table VDistribution of CT scan findings by laterality

CT TAP	Right colon	Left colon	Total
Extension to neighboring organs	1 (3,7%)	7 (8,9%)	8 (7,6%)
Liver metastases	2 (7,4%)	15 (19,2%)	17 (16,2%)
Lung and bone metastases, carcinosis	0	0	0

*TAP CT: thoracoabdomino-pelvic computed tomography

For the right colon group, the most frequent tumor location on TAP CT was at the expense of the right colonic angle in 41% of cases, with the other locations detailed in the following figure (Figure 4).

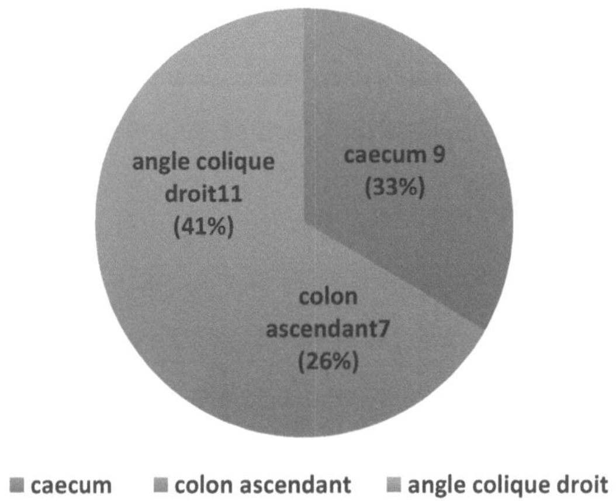

Figure 4Distribution of tumour locations in the right colon on CT scan

For the left colon group, the tumor was located in the sigmoid in 65% of cases, with the other locations detailed in the following figure (Figure 5).

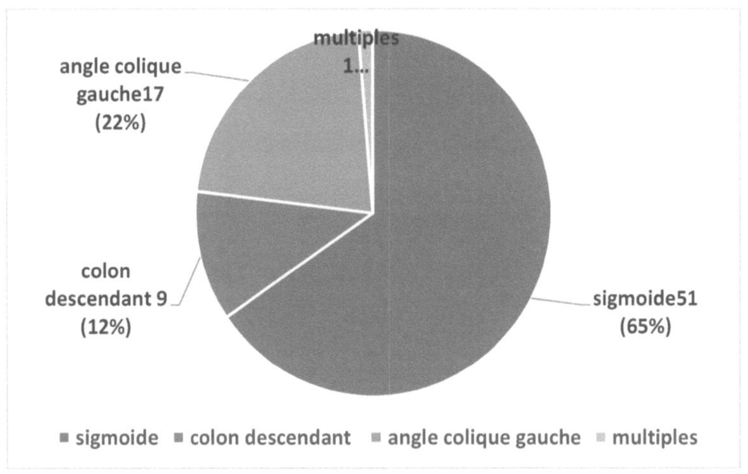

Figure 5Distribution of tumor locations in the left colon on CT scan

1.2.2.3. Liver MRI

Among 17 patients with liver metastases on CT, liver MRI was performed only in 4 patients with left colon tumors.

1.2.2.4. Tumor markers

Carcinoembryonic antigen (CEA) was requested in 19 patients (18%). The distribution according to location is detailed in Table VI :

Table VIDistribution of tumor markers according to tumor laterality

ACE	Right colon	Left colon	Total
Fact	5 (18,5%)	14(17,9%)	19(18%)
Positive	4(80%)	9(64,3%)	13(68,4%)
Negative	1(20%)	5(35,7%)	6(31,6%)

*ACE: Carcinoembryonic antigen

1.2.3. Biological profile (hemoglobin and albumin)

All patients had a complete blood count (CBC). The mean hemoglobinemia in our population was 10.4 mg/dl. Albuminemia was requested in only 56 patients (53.3%), and showed hypo albuminemia in 42.8% of cases. The breakdown by location is shown in Table VII.

Table VIIDistribution of hemoglobulinemia and albuminemia by tumor location

Variable	Right colon	Left colon	Total
Mean hemoglobin mg/dl	10,6 (+/- 2,1)	10,8 (+/- 1,6)	10,4
Anemia (hb<10 mg/dl)	10 (37%)	25 (32%)	35 (33,3%)

| Mean albumin g/l | 32,5 (+/- 4,2) | 34 (+/- 4,3) | 33,6 |
| Hypo albuminemia (<35mg/l) | 5 /11(45,5%) | 19/45 (42,2%) | 24/56 (42,8%) |

1.2.4. Preparing for surgery

Preoperative transfusion was used in 35 cases (33.3%), and parenteral nutrition in 10 cases (9.5%). The distribution according to laterality is detailed in Table VIII. Colonic preparation was performed in 22 patients (28.2%) with left colon tumors.

Table VIIIDistribution of surgical preparation elements according to laterality

Variable	Right colon	Left colon	Total
Preoperative transfusion	10 (37%)	25 (32%)	35 (33,3%)
Parenteral nutrition	5 (18,5%)	5 (6,4%)	10 (9,5%)

1.3. OPERATING CHARACTERISTICS

1.3.1. Circumstances of surgery

Surgery was scheduled in 54 cases (51.4%) and performed on an emergency basis in 51 cases (48.6%). The distribution according to laterality is detailed in table IX.

Table IXDistribution of surgery circumstances according to tumor laterality

Surgery background	Right colon	Left colon	Total
Cold	14 (51,9%)	40(51,3%)	54 (51,4%)

| In a hurry | 13 (48,1%) | 38 (48,7%) | 51(48,6%) |

1.3.2. Surgical approach

All patients undergoing emergency surgery (51 (48.6%)) underwent conventional surgery. For scheduled procedures, the approach was laparoscopic in 18 patients (33.3%), including 5 (19%) with right-colon tumors and 13 (17%) with left-colon tumors. The conventional approach was chosen in 36 patients (66.6%), of whom 22 (81%) had right-colon tumors and 65 (83%) had left-colon tumors.

1.3.3. Intraoperative exploration

Intraoperative exploration revealed 13 cases of ascites of low abundance (negative cytology), 15 cases of hepatic metastases, and locoregional invasion in 16 cases, which did not contraindicate monobloc resection. Other intraoperative findings are detailed in the following table (Table X).

Table XBreakdown of intraoperative findings by tumor laterality

Recognition (n(%))	Right colon	Left colon	Total
Ascites*	3 (11,1%)	10 (12,8%)	13 (12,4%)
Liver metastases	2 (7,4%)	13 (16,6%)	15 (14,2%)
Size			
>3 cm	21 (77,7%)	64 (82%)	85 (80,9%)
>4cm	12 (44,4%)	47 (60,2%)	59 (56,2%)
>5 cm	9 (33,3%)	17 (21,8%)	26 (24,7%)
Locoregional invasion	2 (7,4%)	14 (17,9%)	16 (15,2%)
Occlusive tumor	7 (25,9%)	26 (33,3%)	33 (31,4%)
Generalized peritonitis	1 (3,7%)	3 (3,8%)	4 (3,8%)

| **Superinfected tumor** | 3 (11,1%) | 19 (24,3%) | 22 (20,9%) |

* low abundance with negative cytology

1.3.4. Type of operation

For the right colon group, all patients had a carcinological right colectomy. Two patients did not have immediate restoration of continuity and had an ileostomy because of occlusion with a very distended small bowel in one case and for generalized peritonitis in the other.

For the left colon, the surgical procedure was a low segmental resection in more than half the cases. Three patients underwent colectomy after proximal colostomy: two with low segmental resection and one with true left hemi colectomy. Other surgical procedures performed are summarized in Table XI. Twenty-nine patients did not have immediate restoration of digestive continuity. Ostomy indications for this left colon group were peritonitis in 11 patients (38%) and occlusion in 18 patients (62%).

Table XISurgical treatment for cancer of the left colon

Gesture	Frequency	Percentage
True left hemi colectomy	11	14,1%
High segmental colectomy	10	12,8%
Low segmental colectomy (LSC)**	43	55,1%
Total colectomy	14	17,9%

* A patient after a near upstream colostomy
** two patients after a near upstream stoma

For associated resection procedures, 13 patients underwent Wedge-type hepatic metastasectomies in 7 cases, and regulated hepatectomy, removing 1 or 2 segments, in 6 cases.

1.3.5. Duration of intervention

The average duration of the procedure was 139.5 minutes, with extremes of 75 and 280 minutes (Table XII).

Table XII Duration of surgery according to tumour location

	Right colon	Left colon	Total
Duration of intervention (min) Average [min - max]	139,4 [75 - 180]	180 [90 - 280]	169,5 [75 - 280]

1.4. POST-OPERATIVE

Postoperative follow-up was straightforward in 58 cases, with a mean postoperative stay of 6.68 days (Table XIII). Post-operative mortality was 0.

Table XIIIElements of the operative follow-up according to tumor location

Variables	Right colon n(%)	Left colon	Total
Simple suites	16 (59,3%)	42 (53,8%)	58 (55,2%)
Overall morbidity	11 (48,7%)	36 (46,2%)	47 (44,8%)
Anastomotic fistula	2 (7%)	8 (10,2%)	10 (9,5%)

Post-operative stay (d)			
Average	5,12	7,23	6,68
[min - max]	[3-7]	[3-18]	[3-18]

1.5. ANATOMOPATHOLOGICAL DATA :

Invasive adenocarcinoma was found in all cases, the tumor was classified T3 or higher in 95 cases (90%), N+ in 60 cases (57%) (Table XIV).

Table XIV Anatomopathological characteristics by tumor location

Observation / location		Right colon	Left colon	Total
T	**Tis***	0	0	0
	T1	1 (3,7%)	1 (1,3%)	2 (1,9%)
	T2	4 (14,8%)	4 (5,1%)	8 (7,6%)
	T3	12 (44,4%)	41 (52,6%)	53 (50,4%)
	T4	10 (37%)	32 (41%)	42 (40%)
N	**N0**	13 (48,1%)	32 (48,1%)	45 (42,8%)
	N1	11 (40,7%)	28 (35,9%)	39 (37,1%)
	N2	3 (11,1%)	18 (23%)	21 (20%)
M	**M0**	25 (92,6%)	62 (79,5%)	87 (82,8%)
	M+	2 (7,4%)	16 (20,5%)	18 (17,1%)
TNM stage	**Cis****	0	0	0
	I	4 (14,8%)	3 (3,8%)	7 (6,6%)
	II	9 (33,3%)	29 (37,2%)	38 (36,2%)
	III	12 (44,4%)	30 (38,5%)	42 (40%)
	IV	2 (7,4%)	16 (20,5%)	18 (17,1%)
Vascular emboli		11 (40,7%)	31 (39,7%)	42 (40%)

| Lymphatic emboli | 12 (44,4%) | 29 (37,2%) | 41 (39%) |
| Perineural swelling | 18 (66,7%) | 42 (53,8%) | 60 (57,1%) |

*Tis: Tumor in situ
**Cis: Carcinoma in situ

1.6.   ADJUVANT TREATMENT

Adjuvant chemotherapy was administered to 72 patients (68.5%): 17 patients (63%) had right-colon tumors and 55 (70.5%) had left-colon tumors.

1.7.   SURVIVAL

For the right colon group, overall survival was 57% at 3 years and 52% at 5 years. For the left colon group, survival was 67.6% at 3 years and 56.5% at 5 years (Figure 6).

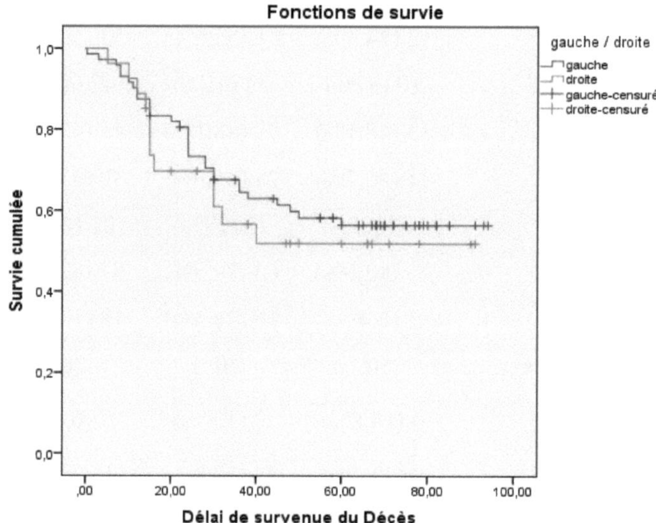

Figure 6Overall survival by tumour location

Recurrence-free survival for the right colon group was 56% at 3

years and 51% at 5 years. For the left colon group, it was 60.3% at 3 years
and 54.1% at 5 years (Figure 7).

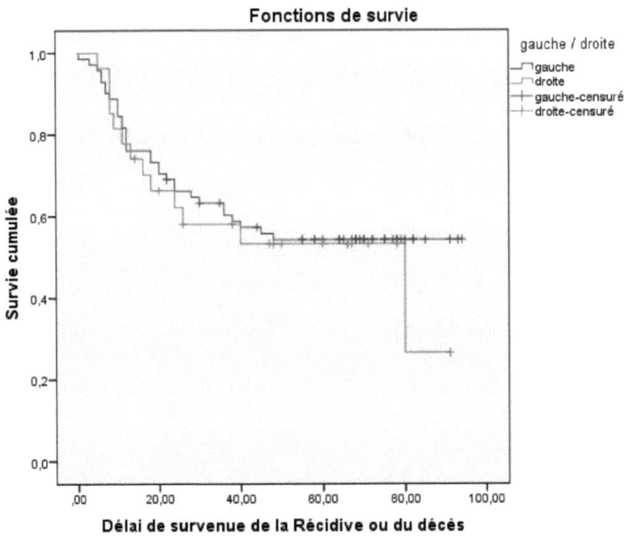

Figure 7Recurrence-free survival by tumor location

2. ANALYTICAL STUDY

2.1. COMPARISON OF DIFFERENT PARAMETERS ACCORDING TO LATERALITY

* Epidemiological characteristics

Comparison of epidemiological characteristics according to tumor laterality revealed a single "Diabetes" variable statistically more frequent in the right colon cancer group (Table XV).

Table XVComparison of epidemiological characteristics by laterality

	Right colon	**Left colon**	**P value**
Gender	H = 59,3% F= 40,7%	H = 46,2% F= 53,8%	0,17
Age	65.48 years	65.06 years	0,89
Tobacco	No = 44.4% Yes = 55.6%	No = 61.5% Yes = 38.5%	0,09
Alcohol	No: 85.2% Yes = 14.8%	No = 83.3% Yes = 16.7%	0,54
Obesity	No: 66.7%. Yes: 33.3%	No = 49 Yes = 51	0,18
Diabetes	No = 66.7% of the total Yes: 33.3%	No = 84.4% Yes = 15.6%	**0,045**
HTA*	No = 70.5% Yes = 29.5%	No = 63 Yes = 37	0,309
Heart disease	No = 92.6% Yes = 7.4%	No = 92.3% Yes = 7.7%.	0,66
Pneumopathy	No = 96.3% Yes = 3.7%.	No = 98.7% Yes = 1.3%	0,45

- Circumstances of discovery

Comparison of the circumstances of discovery according to tumor laterality concluded that the presence of an abdominal mass on clinical examination is statistically significantly more frequent on the right side (Table XVI).

Table XVIComparison of circumstances of discovery according to tumor laterality

	Right colon	Left colon	P value
Abdominal pain	85,2%	76,9%	0,27
Transit disorders	66,6%	62,8%	0,19
AEG*	59,8%	53,3%	0,6
Lower digestive hemorrhage	11,1%	16,7%	0,36
Abdominal mass	29,6%	15,4%	**0,04**
Revealing Complication	29,6%	34,6%	0,411
Occlusion	3,7%	5,1%	0,61
Peritonitis	14,7%	9%	0,3
Localized defense			

* AEG: Impaired general condition

- Operating data

Comparison of operative data by laterality showed that operative time was significantly longer for left-sided colon cancers. In addition, the incidence of liver metastases was higher in the left colon cancer group (Table XVII).

Table XVIIComparison of operative data by tumor laterality

	Right colon	Left colon	P value
Scheduled surgery	51,9%	48,87%	0,42
Emergency surgery	48,1%	48,7%	0.58
Tumor size			
> 3 cm	77,7%	82%	0,36
> 4 cm	44,4%	60,2%	0.46
> 5cm	33,3%	21,8%	0.38
Locoregional invasion	7,4%	17,9%	0,15
Ascites*	11,1%	12,8%	0,56
Liver metastases	7,4%	20,8%	**0,045**
Intervention time	156 min	178 min	**0,042**
Overall morbidity	40,7%	47,4%	0,35
Anastomotic fistula	7,4%	12,8%	0,35

*low abundance

- Pathological data

Comparison of pathological data showed no significant differences between right and left colon cancer. The T1 and T2 groups were not compared due to lack of numbers. (Table XVIII).

Table XVIIIComparison of anatomopathological data by tumor laterality

	Right colon	Left colon	P value

T3	44,4%	52,6%	0,12
T4	37%	41%	0,9
N +*	52%	45%	0,3
Perineural swelling	66,7%	53,8%	0,17
Vascular emboli	40,7%	39,7%	0,55
Lymphatic emboli	44,4%	37,2%	0,32

*N+: lymph node metastases

- Overall survival and recurrence-free survival

Comparison of overall and recurrence-free survival showed no significant differences according to tumor location (Table XIX) (Figure 8,9).

Painting XIX Assessment of survival according to tumor laterality

	Right colon		Left colon		P value
	3 years	5 years	3 years	5 years	
Overall survival	56,6%	51,9%	67,6%	56,5%	0,571
Recurrence-free survival	56%	51,2%	63,3%	54,1%	0,631

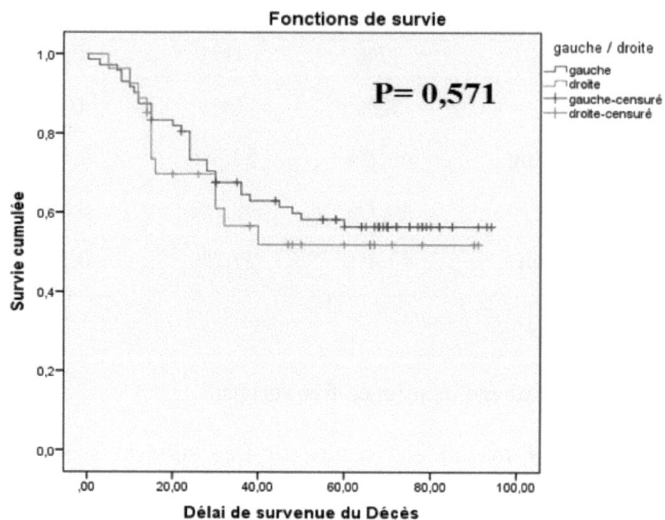

Figure 8 Comparison of overall survival by tumor location

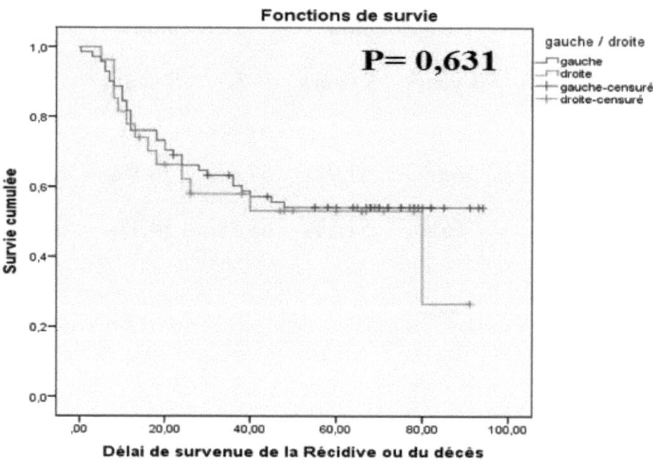

Figure 9Comparison of recurrence-free survival by tumor location

2.2. STUDY OF OVERALL SURVIVAL AS A FUNCTION OF VARIOUS POSITIVE PARAMETERS

Our univariate analytical study found common poor prognostic factors (right colon group and left colon group) on overall survival (Table XX).

In addition, our sample showed specific factors according to laterality summarized in Tables XXI and XXII.

Table XX Study of overall survival according to significant factors

Parameters	Right colon		Left colon	
	5-year survival	P-value	5-year survival	P-value
Age	<= 70 years: 75.6% >70 years: 20%.	**0,029**	<= 70 years: 67.8% >70 years: 37.1%	**0,005**
HTA*	No : 68,3% Yes: 25%.	**0,046**	No: 63.7% No: 63.7% No: 63.7% No: 63.7% No: 63.7 Yes: 38.2%	**0,018**
ASA	I : 88,9% II: 36.7% OF SALES	**0,041**	I : 65,4% II: 59.1% III: 0% OF SALES	**<0,001**
Tumor size (mm)**	No: 100%. Yes: 37.8%	**0,023**	No: 69 Yes : 46.5%	**0,049**
Perforated tumor	No : 59,1% Yes: 0%.	**0,022**	No : 60,6% Yes : 43.8%	**0,049**
Perineural swelling	No : 77,8% Yes : 38.5%	**0,032**	No : 76,8% Yes: 35.9%	**0,002**
Venous emboli	No: 60.3% Yes: 27.3%	**0,05**	No: 67.4% Yes : 36.5%	**0,02**
Lymphatic emboli	No: 72.2% Yes: 23.4%	**0,007**	No: 67 Yes: 35.8%	**0,005**

* HTA: high blood pressure

 **Tumor size: > 3 cm for right colon and > 5 for left colon

Table XXIOverall survival study based on significant factors specific to the right colon

Parameters	Survival to 5 years	P-value
Peritonitis	No: 53.9% Yes: 0%.	0,03
Locoregional invasion	No: 56.2% Yes: 0%.	0,009
T4	Yes: 13 No: 73.9%	0,004

Table XXIIStudy of overall survival as a function of significant factors specific to the left colon

Parameters	Survival to 5 years	P-value
Intraoperative metastases	No : 66,9% Yes: 0%.	<0,001
N+*	No: 66 Yes: 41.3%	0,029

* N+: lymph node metastases

2.3. STUDY OF RECURRENCE-FREE SURVIVAL AS A FUNCTION OF DIFFERENT POSITIVE PARAMETERS

The study of recurrence-free survival found common poor prognostic factors for patients with right and left colon cancer, which are summarized in Table XXIII.

In addition, our sample showed specific factors according to laterality, which are summarized in Tables XXIV and XXV.

Table XXIIIStudy of recurrence-free survival according to significant common factors

	Right colon		Left colon	
	SSR at 5 years	**P-value**	**SSR at 5 years**	**P-value**
Age	<= 70 years: 76.5% >70 years: 20%.	**0,021**	<= 70 years: 65.7% >70 years: 34.6%	**0,011**
Tumor size	No: 100%. Yes: 40%.	**0,025**	No: 70%. Yes: 42	**0,016**
Locoregional invasion	No: 56.2% Yes: 0%.	**0,009**	No: 58 Yes: 30%.	**0,045**
Perforated tumor	No: 60.4% Yes: 0%.	**0,037**	No: 59.2% Yes: 37.5%	**0,037**
Perineural swelling	No : 77,8% Yes: 42	**0,048**	No: 76.2% Yes: 33.4%	**0,001**
Lymphatic emboli	No: 72.7%. Yes: 26	**0,009**	No: 63 Yes: 37.3%	**0,022**

*Tumor size: > 3 cm for the right colon and > 5 cm for the left colon

Table XXIVStudy of recurrence-free survival as a function of significant factors specific to the right colon

Parameters	SSR at 5 years	P-value

Peritonitis	No: 55.2%	**0,022**
	Yes: 0%.	
T4	Yes: 21.2%	**0,009**
	No: 76	

Table XXVStudy of recurrence-free survival according to significant factors specific to the left colon

Parameters	SSR at 5 years	P-value
Scheduled/emergency surgery	Cold: 66.4%	**0,049**
	Emergency: 41.3	
Metastases	No: 63.4%	**<0,001**
	Yes : 11.1%	
ASA score	I : 62,7%	**<0,001**
	II: 56.6%	
	III: 0% OF SALES	
N+*	No: 63.4%	**0,045**
	Yes: 41.3%	

* N+: lymph node metastases

DISCUSSION

The distinction between right and left colon cancer remains controversial. In our country, few studies have discussed the influence of tumour location on carcinological prognosis, with recurrence rates estimated at between 15% and 30%, irrespective of location. (13). A better understanding of the epidemiological and clinical features and prognostic factors of each tumour site could provide the information needed to improve therapeutic management and prognosis.

Indeed, the practical interest of our study is to identify the epidemiological, clinical and histological characteristics of each tumor location and their impact on survival and prognosis.

1. ANSWERS TO OUR RESEARCH QUESTIONS

a) **Main objective**: To assess the impact of right or left colon cancer location on patient prognosis after curative surgery.

Our sample showed no significant differences in terms of overall and recurrence-free survival.

For the right colon, overall survival is estimated at 56.6% at 3 years and 51.9% at 5 years; for the left colon, it is 67.6% at 3 years and 56.6% at 5 years.

Recurrence-free survival was estimated at 56% at 3 years and 51.2% at 5 years for the right colon; and 63.3% at 3 years and 54.1% at 5 years for the left colon.

Although the differences are not significant, the left colon appears to have slightly better overall and recurrence-free survival.

Our analytical study concluded that the common poor prognostic factors on overall survival in a patient with a right or left colon tumor are:

- Age over 70.

- High blood pressure.
- ASA score greater than or equal to II.
- Per-operative finding of a perforated tumour or a large tumour (over 3 cm for the right colon or over 5 cm for the left colon).
- An anatomopathological examination showing peri-nervous sheathing, vascular and/or lymphatic emboli.

In addition to the common factors already mentioned, our sample showed specific factors according to laterality; on the one hand, the intra-operative finding of peritonitis or locoregional invasion and a pathological examination showing a T4 tumor are poor prognostic factors in patients with right-sided colon cancer. On the other hand, the presence of liver metastases and lymph node involvement on pathological examination are considered poor prognostic factors for overall survival in patients with left-sided colon cancer.

Regarding recurrence-free survival, our study concluded that the common poor prognostic factors for patients with right or left colon cancer are :

- Age over 70.
- Per-operative finding of a perforated or large tumor (greater than 3 cm for the right colon and greater than 5 cm for the left colon).
- Pathological examination reveals peri-nervous sheathing or vascular and/or lymphatic emboli.

In addition, other statistically significant factors of poor prognosis on recurrence-free survival specific to each location were identified. Factors specific to the right side were the intraoperative finding of peritonitis and the presence of a tumour greater than T3 on pathological examination. For the left side, the specific factors are: ASA score greater than II, intraoperative finding of hepatic metastases, surgery in an emergency context and the presence of lymph node invasion on pathological examination.

b) **Secondary objective**: Evaluate the epidemiological, clinical and histological profile of each tumor site.

Our study showed in a statistically significant way that :

- Diabetes is more common in the right colon cancer group.
- The presence of an abdominal mass on clinical examination is more frequent in tumors of the right colon.
- Tumors of the left colon are more likely to be associated with synchronous liver metastases than tumors of the right colon.
- Surgery time is longer for left-sided colon cancers.

In addition, our comparative study yielded non-statistically significant findings, which are:

- Abdominal pain and diarrhea appear to be more frequent in right-sided colon cancers, while constipation and digestive hemorrhage appear to be more frequent on the left side.
- Cancer of the right colon appeared to be more frequently complicated by superinfection or peritonitis, whereas cancer of the left colon was more frequently complicated by occlusion.
- Cancer of the left colon appears to have a greater potential for invasion of its wall (T), whereas cancer of the right colon appears to be more frequently accompanied by lymph node metastases and histological elements of poor prognosis (EPN, EV and El).

2. LIMITATIONS OF OUR STUDY

The main limitation of our study is its retrospective nature, which induces the risk of several biases. On the one hand, missing data and different operative protocols from one operator to another induce a patient selection bias. On the other hand, the socio-economic level of the population consulting our hospital and the conditions of hospitalization also represent a source of selection bias, given the mono-centric nature of the study.

In addition, the limited number of patients, especially in the right colon cancer group, could influence the results of our study by reducing its power.

Moreover, our population is not homogeneous, given the inclusion of colon cancers of different clinical presentations (elective surgery, emergency surgery) and tumor stages.

In addition, the multivariate study of poor prognostic factors on overall survival and recurrence-free survival was not carried out due to deficiencies in the application of its criteria, notably the verification of the proportional risks hypothesis and the limited number of patients in the subgroups.

On the other hand, molecular features of the tumor, such as MSS/MSI phenotype, BRAF, KRAS and CIMP mutations, which currently represent important prognostic elements in the literature, were not evaluated in our study. These missing data could help us to better understand the prognostic impact of molecular markers on colon cancers according to their sites in our population.

3. BIBLIOGRAPHICAL RESEARCH AND VALIDATION OF OUR RESULTS

3.1. Main objective: Impact of right or left location of primary adenocarcinoma on cancer prognosis

3.1.1. Overall survival

Several studies have investigated the overall survival of colon cancers according to their location.

Benedix et al, including 8297 patients operated on for right-sided colon adenocarcinoma versus 9344 patients operated on for left-sided colon adenocarcinoma, concluded that left-sided localization had a statistically proven better 5-year survival (71% vs. 67%) P=0.01. However, patient survival was influenced by disease stage (OR=2; p<0.01), ASA score (OR=1.72; p<0.01) and extended resections (OR=1.81; p<0.01), which were more common in the right colon.(14).

In 2011, the American epidemiological study, based on the SEER (Surveillance, Epidemiology and End Results) program database, included 77978 patients operated on between 1988 and 2003(15). It concluded that median survival was better for patients operated on for adenocarcinoma of the left colon, with a significant difference (78 vs. 89 months; p<0.001). This difference was significant in the multivariate study only for stages III and IV (p=0.01; HR= 1.12 [1.06 to 1.8]).

These findings were reinforced by the meta-analysis and review of the literature by Petrelli et al, analyzing 66 studies made from 1995 to 2016 and including 1,437,846 patients operated on for colonic adenocarcinoma, reported a better prognosis of left localization in terms of overall survival with a statistically significant difference (OR= 0.82 [0.79 ;0.84] ; p<0.001) independent of race, tumor stage, adjuvant therapy and year of study(16).

Warschow et al. in 2016 challenged these findings. Using the

Surveillance, Epidemiology, and End Results (SEER) database (2004-2012), he identified 91,416 patients with stage I to III colon cancer (51,937 right colon cancers and 39,479 left colon cancers) (17). In univariate analysis, patients with left-sided cancer had better cancer-specific survival (HR = 1.26, 95% CI: 1.21-1.30, P < 0.001) than patients with right-sided cancer. However, after matching, the prognosis for right-sided cancers was better in terms of overall survival (HR = 0.92, 95% CI: 0.89 - 0.94, P < 0.001) and cancer-specific survival (HR = 0.90, 95% CI: 0.87 - 0.93, P < 0.001). This difference is more pronounced for stages I and II. This calls into question the paradigm of previous studies asserting better survival in patients with left-sided colon cancer.

More recently in 2019, a Korean study by Yang MK et al included 2329 patients after matching eight variables (age, sex, T stage, N stage, histological grade, presence of lymphovascular/peri-neuronal invasion and microsatellite instability status) (18). This study showed that overall survival was statistically inferior for patients with stage III right colon cancer (HR, 1.561; 95% CI, 0.967-2.522; P = 0.068).

Also in 2019, a Mayo Clinic study compared the overall survival of 15880 patients with left-sided colon cancer versus 7570 patients with right-sided colon cancer(19) . It concluded that left-sided localization was associated with statistically better median survival, with a significant difference (93 months vs. 76.6 months; p<0.00001).

Other recent studies have shown no significant difference in overall survival, such as the 2019 study by Jasmine Lizette Gowarty et al. and the prospective study published in 2020 by Metin Keskin et al. (20). However, these two studies have different inclusion criteria, notably the inclusion of tumors extending to the left colonic angle in the right colon tumor group.

The Tunisian multicenter study, presented at the 2021 congress of the

Tunisian Colorectal Cancer Association (ATCCR), showed that survival was significantly diminished by tumor location on the left (p=0.05). This was explained by the presence of more metastatic forms in the left colon group (56 patients or 19.5%) compared with the right colon group (38 patients or 12%), with a difference at the limit of significance (p=0.06).

Thus, most studies affirm the better prognosis of left colon cancers in terms of overall survival, especially for advanced stages of the disease, while for early stages, right colon cancer appears to have a better prognosis.

In our series, tumors of the left colon were associated with better 3-year and 5-year overall survival than those of the right colon, with a non-significant p value (p=0.571). The non-significant difference could be explained by the limited number of patients in the right colon cancer group and the greater number of metastatic forms in the left colon cancer group.

3.1.2. Recurrence-free survival

Tumor recurrence at 5 years varies in the literature from 6 to 25% depending on tumor stage (21,22). This recurrence frequently occurred in the first two years after curative surgery(21). Several studies have compared recurrence-free survival according to tumour location.

A Japanese study by Moritani et al published in 2013, compared recurrence-free survival in 820 patients (399 patients with right colon cancer and 421 with left colon cancer) over a mean follow-up period of 55.8 ± 34.9 months(23). There were no significant differences in five-year disease-free survival between the two populations (right 88.6%; left 89.4%; P = 0.231). Subgroup analyses showed that patients with stage I right-sided colon cancer had a significantly better 5-year recurrence-free survival rate than those with left-sided cancer (100 vs. 95.2%, P = 0.034).

In 2015, a Korean study analyzed 1,632 patients operated on for non-metastatic colon adenocarcinoma at the National Cancer Center in Korea between January 2001 and December 2009(24). It compared recurrence-free survival rates according to tumour location. It showed a significantly shorter time to locoregional recurrence for patients with right-sided colon cancer (HR = 2.35; p < 0.001), with a statistically significant difference in locoregional recurrence for the same group (8.5% vs. 4.1%).

Then a Chinese study by QinQ et al was published in 2017, comparing 317 patients operated on for right colon tumors with 310 for left colon tumors(25). Right-sided colon cancer had a statistically higher incidence of recurrence than left-sided cancer (30.6% vs. 23.2%, P = 0.037). Subgroup analysis showed that patients with left-sided colon cancer had significantly better 5-year recurrence-free survival rates than those with stage III right-sided cancer (64.3% vs. 46.8%, P = 0.002). This difference was not noted in stage I and II disease.

A prospective study by Lee JM et al. published in 2019, included 1912 patients operated on for colon tumors(26). In univariate analysis, recurrence-free survival was similar at 5 years for right and left colon cancer. This was also noted for stages I and II disease. However, for stage III patients, an adjusted Cox regression analysis indicated that right colon cancer patients had a higher risk of cancer-specific mortality (HR, 1.75; 95% CI, 1.07-2.86; P = 0.024) and recurrence (HR, 1.78; 95% CI, 1.22-2.60; P = 0.003). In addition, right colon cancer was an independent predictor of peritoneal recurrence (HR, 1.86; 95% CI, 1.05-3.29; P = 0.031) in stage III patients.

However, in 2020, a study including 990 patients by the Mayo Clinic team called into question the above findings for non-advanced stages (stage II) (19). The postoperative recurrence rate for cancer of the left colon (descending colon, sigmoid colon) was higher than for cancer of the right colon (coecum, ascending colon, transverse colon) (OR 2.191, 95% CI 1.091-4.400, P = 0.027). In the COX survival factor analysis for colon cancer, the left side was one of the independent risk factors (relative risk 5.377, 95% CI 0.216-0.88, P = 0.02).

A recent study published in 2O22, included 1017 patients who underwent curative colectomy for stage I-III colon cancer at Shang-Ho Hospital in Taiwan, between August 2008 and December 2019. It did not show the same findings as those of the Mayo Clinic. In subgroup analysis, this study showed that right-sided colon cancer was associated with a shorter time to recurrence than left-sided stage II colon cancer (HR 2.36, 95% confidence interval 1.24-4.48, p < 0.01). Thus, right-sided stage II colon cancer was an independent risk factor for recurrence.

Our sample showed no significant differences in terms of recurrence-free survival. However, it appears that tumors in the left colon have a better prognosis. Indeed, recurrence-free survival for the left colon is estimated at 63.3% at 3 years and 54.1% at 5 years. For the right colon, it is estimated at 56% at 3 years and 51.2% at 5 years. The statistically insignificant difference could be explained by the advanced tumour stage of the left colon group at the time of diagnosis.

Thus, in terms of recurrence-free survival according to the laterality of colonic cancers, the results are divergent: some studies report a lower recurrence rate for left colon cancers of all stages, while others, by analyzing subgroups, have shown that early-stage right colon cancers have a better recurrence-free survival. On the other hand, other studies have found contrary data. This divergence in results from different studies could be explained by genetic and environmental factors.

3.2. Secondary objective: evaluation of the epidemiological, clinical and histological profile of each tumor site.

3.2.1. Epidemiological and clinical factors

- **Age :**

Advanced age is no longer considered a contraindication to colonic surgery(27). This is explained by the development of perioperative resuscitation and the widespread use of minimally invasive surgery (28).

Advanced age is correlated with a decrease in overall survival and recurrence-free survival according to several studies such as those by Ronald C, Chapuis and Parc HC(29), (30), (31).

With regard to the impact of laterality, and depending on the epidemiological profile of the series, right-sided localization is characterized by an advanced age of patients. This may be explained by the less eloquent symptomatology of right-sided cancers, characterized by a wider lumen, which delays diagnosis and thus poorens prognosis. (32) (33) (34).

In our series, an age greater than 70 years was associated with reduced overall survival and recurrence-free survival in colon cancer patients in the 2 "right and left" groups. Also, Our study showed that patients with right colon cancer are older, but this difference was not statistically proven, this could be explained by the small sample size of the right colon group.

- **Gender :**

Some studies claim that female gender is associated with reduced survival(24,31). Others have shown that male gender is an independent poor prognostic factor for overall survival and recurrence-free survival

(29,35) . However, the Radespiel-Tröger study, including 641 patients operated on for colonic adenocarcinoma, showed that there was no significant difference in terms of 5-year recurrence-free survival between women and men, irrespective of location (77% vs. 80%, p=0.06) (36).

With regard to laterality, data from the literature have shown divergent results in terms of sex distribution according to tumor location, with a tendency for greater female frequency in the right colon group (34) (37) (38).

Indeed, to date, there is a lack of statistically solid evidence to confirm the variation in tumor location according to gender.

In our series, male or female sex did not appear to be a factor in poor prognosis. Our series showed a male predominance of right colon cancer, with no significant difference.

- **Obesity:**

Obesity is currently a public health problem. The relative risk of developing colorectal cancer in obese patients is 4.9(39). The impact of obesity on survival and recurrence has rarely been analyzed. A 2013 Mayo Clinic study revealed an association between body mass index (BMI) and colon cancer prognosis(40). Indeed, obese patients with a BMI greater than 35 kg/m2 had significantly diminished overall survival with an increased rate of cancer recurrence. Furthermore, obese men in classes 2 and 3 (BMI ≥ 35.0 kg/m(2)) had a statistically significant reduction in disease-free survival (relative risk [HR], 1.16; 95% CI confidence interval, [1.01-1.33]; P = 0.0297) compared with patients in class 1.

Very few data are available on the correlation of obesity with tumor laterality. Brulé et al in 2015 found a statistical association between obesity and left-sided colon cancer (41).

In our sample, obesity did not appear to be a poor prognostic factor.

- **Tobacco and alcohol:**

Smoking and excessive alcohol consumption are recognized risk factors for developing colorectal cancer. The association of these two factors with recurrence and overall survival after colorectal surgery is increasingly being discussed(42-44).

For the impact of laterality, the majority of the literature has not shown a proven relationship. A few articles have reported associations, such as the study by Qin Q et al, which showed an association of left-sided colon cancer with duration of smoking(25). This association was not found for cancers of the right colon.

The study of our sample showed no correlation between smoking and alcoholism and tumour location.

- **Comorbidities and ASA score:**

Several studies have concluded that the presence of comorbidities with a high ASA score adversely affects survival(45-48). However, ASA scores are assigned using several patient-specific factors, including nutritional status and medical history, which were themselves identified as poor prognostic factors for colorectal cancer. This induces a confounding bias in these studies. Yanic R et Al concluded that arterial hypertension, cardiac disease, arthritis and chronic lung disease are associated with a significant decrease in 2-year overall survival (p=0.0007) irrespective of location (45). Stein KB's systematic review and meta-analysis showed a significant increase in specific long-term mortality and 5-year recurrence in diabetic patients (32% mortality, 95% CI: 1.24, 1.41) (49). Recent studies have demonstrated a difference according to location, and have shown that the presence of comorbidities such as diabetes, hypertension, dyslipidemia and heart failure are more frequent on the right side(50) (33). However, Tapia Rico et al. noted a greater frequency of diabetes in left-sided colon cancer(34).

In our series, arterial hypertension and ASA score greater than or equal to II were identified as poor prognostic factors on overall survival common to both groups.

3.2.2. Circumstances of surgery and intraoperative findings

- Circumstances of discovery excluding complications :

Analysis of the literature has shown significant differences according to the circumstances of discovery of uncomplicated colonic cancer in relation to laterality (129). On the one hand, right-colon tumors have an unspecific symptomatology such as abdominal pain, weight loss and anemia. On the other hand, left colon tumours cause transit disorders and haemorrhage(130,131).

In our study, tumors of the left colon presented mainly with digestive hemorrhage and/or constipation, whereas those of the right colon presented with diarrhea and abdominal pain, but with no significant difference.

- Emergency surgery

Several studies have reported a reduction in overall and recurrence-free survival in patients undergoing emergency surgery, irrespective of tumour location. A study published in 2006 by Burton et al showed that the 3-year survival rate for patients undergoing emergency surgery was 48.21% (95% CI: 25.22-67.94%), compared with 78.72% (95% CI: 71.55-84.28%) for patients undergoing scheduled surgery.(51).

In our series, the comparative study showed no significant difference between emergency surgery and tumor location. However, emergency surgery is a poor prognostic factor for recurrence-free survival in left-sided colon cancers.

- Complicated forms :

Complicated forms are associated with a poor prognosis in terms of survival, according to several studies. A study published in 2009 by Cheynel et al showed that the five-year cumulative local recurrence rate was higher for perforated cancers (15.7%) than for uncomplicated cancers (7.8%; P = 0.021) (52). A Korean study by Yik-Hong Ho et al concluded in univariate and multivariate analysis that occlusion and perforation had a statistically significant negative impact on recurrence-free survival, with an HR equal to 2.5 irrespective of tumor stage, histological grade and presence of vascular emboli.(53). Other recent studies have confirmed these results, such as Yang K M's study published in May 2022(54).

Tumor size is associated with poorer overall survival and recurrence-free survival in several studies(55-57). The study by Liang et al, published in 2021, concluded that tumor size greater than 5 cm was associated with significantly lower 5-year overall survival and relapse-free survival (OS: 63.5% vs. 75.2%, P < 0.001; RFS: 59.5% vs. 72.4%, P < 0.001). (58). Also in 2021, the study by Alese et al deduced that the prognostic impact of tumor size was strongly associated with survival to stage III disease. This hazard ratio evolves in the same direction as tumour size(59).

Concerning laterality, cancer of the left colon is more frequently manifested by acute intestinal obstruction. This could be explained by the reduced diameter of the distal colon(60). On the other hand, tumors of the right colon had a larger tumor size, which explains their discovery on the occasion of an abdominal mass(61) (62).

In our study, the intraoperative finding of a perforated tumour or a large tumour (greater than 3 cm for the right colon or greater than 5 cm for the left colon) is a poor prognostic factor for overall survival and recurrence-free survival. In addition, it appears that tumors in the left colon are more likely to be complicated by occlusion, while those in the right by septic complications, with no significant difference. In addition, the presence of an abdominal mass is more frequent in right-sided colon cancer, with a statistically proven difference.

- Operating time

The study by Cienfuegos et al showed that operative time was longer for left colon cancers, with a statistically significant difference (146 min vs 165 min; p < 0.001) (22). The Tunisian Colorectal Cancer Association's 2021 multicenter study showed a longer operative time for left colon cancers (176.3 min vs. 187.4; p=0.023).

Our series found the same findings (156 min vs 178min; p=0.042).

3.2.3. Biological factors

Hypoalbuminemia is known to be an independent risk factor for anastomotic loosening(63). Some studies assert that hypoalbuminemia is associated with a reduced survival rate(64,65). The study by Fujii et al showed that the risk of recurrence was significantly increased in cases of hypo albuminemia (33.3% vs. 6.4%; p =0.002) (66).

Some studies have reported that the ratio of neutrophils to lymphocytes is a powerful predictor of survival in patients with colon cancer. This ratio is a combined indicator of inflammation and immunology, and an indicator of response to treatment. The study by Pei-Rong et al showed that a neutrophil/lymphocyte ratio greater than 4 was an unfavorable prognostic factor for recurrence-free survival (HR=4.88;

P<0.01) (67). The study by Mallapa et al revealed that this preoperative ratio, when greater than 5, was an independent risk factor for recurrence (68).

A recent systematic review and meta-analysis published in 2021, showed that a high pre-treatment C-reactive protein (CRP) to albumin ratio was associated with poor overall survival and disease-free survival in colorectal cancer(69). It may serve as a prognostic marker for colorectal cancer in clinical practice. However, this study did not analyze right and left subgroups.

CEA is the reference tumor marker in colorectal cancer. However, its prognostic value in terms of recurrence remains debated (70,71). In the study by Kim et al, an elevated preoperative serum CEA level (≥ 3 ng/mL) is an independent poor prognostic factor on overall survival and recurrence-free survival in patients with stage III colon cancer after curative resection irrespective of tumor location(72).

On the other hand, several studies have shown that patients with adenocarcinoma of the right colon have more anemia than patients with adenocarcinoma of the left colon(22,73). Keeler et al and Dunne et al explained this notion by the larger size of right colon cancers(74) (75).

In our sample, no relationship was reported between the biological factors described above, including hemoglobin level, and overall survival and recurrence-free survival. Furthermore, our study showed no significant differences in terms of biological factors in relation to tumour laterality.

3.2.4. Histological factors

- Tumor stage:

TNM classification is the most important prognostic element, and the best guide to the decision on adjuvant treatment. Several studies have shown that T stage determines the degree of vascular and lymphatic infiltration, and the risk of distant metastases. It also predicts the risk of local and distant recurrence(76,77). In 2008, Quah et al concluded in a study of 448 patients that serosal invasion (T4) increased the risk of death at 5 years by a factor of 3 (p=0.02). (78). These findings were reinforced by the systematic review and meta-analysis by Bockelman et al published in 2015 (79).

Node invasion is an important prognostic factor and the main indication for adjuvant treatment. Several studies have confirmed the poor prognosis of node-positive tumours(24,80,81). The study by Burton et al showed that for a tumor classified as N0, overall survival at 5 years was 75.93%, whereas it was 35.26% for a tumor classified as N2(51). In a study of 716 patients, Ogino et al showed that negative lymph node count was associated with improved survival in colorectal cancer patients, independently of lymphocytic responses to the tumor and tumor molecular characteristics, including MSI, CIMP, LINE-1 hypomethylation and BRAF mutation(82).

The number of lymph nodes removed during lymph node dissection has also been retained as an independent survival factor in colon cancer, independently of lymph node invasion(83) (84).

Moreover, resection margins are a major prognostic factor, a predictor of local recurrence and an indicator of adjuvant therapy(80,85).

For the study of laterality, several studies have found that right colon cancer has an advanced tumor stage compared to left colon cancer, making its prognosis more dismal. In 2017, a study by Lim et al comparing 207 right colon cancer patients with 207 left colon cancer patients showed that right colon cancer had a more advanced N stage, increased tumor size and more lymph nodes removed (86). This study was reinforced by a recent study in 2022 by Yang et al, which showed that right colon cancer had a higher T and N2 stage than left colon cancer(87). Recently, for right colon cancers, some centers have suggested that a more radical curage called complete excision of the right mesocolon could lead to better survival results(88,89).

In our series, the statistically significant poor prognostic factors for overall survival and recurrence-free survival were a T4 tumor for right colon cancer, and lymph node involvement for left colon cancer. In terms of laterality, our series showed no significant differences in terms of tumour stage.

- Histo-pronostic factors:

Several studies have shown that poorly differentiated or undifferentiated tumors are associated with a poor prognosis, as they have a greater risk of parietal invasion, lymph node metastases and distant metastases(90-92). The study by Burton et al showed that 5-year survival fell from 59% for well- or moderately differentiated tumors to 29% for poorly differentiated tumors (p=0.0002) (51).

Histological subtype is an important histoprognostic factor. Studies by Borger et al and O'Connell et al have shown that independent cell adenocarcinomas have a greater risk of vascular and lymphatic invasion, lymph node metastases and distant metastases, resulting in a higher recurrence rate and a poor prognosis.(93) (94).

The presence of tumor emboli in lymphatic and/or vascular structures, and peri-nervous sheathing, are considered predictive of lymph node and distant metastatic dissemination. They are associated with reduced overall survival and recurrence-free survival (95,96). Krasna et al concluded that the incidence of metastases in patients with vascular or neural invasion was more frequent ((60% vs. 17% for vascular invasion (P < 0.0001) and 72.7% vs. 27% for peri-nerve sheathing (P < 0.01)) (97). This study also showed that survival in patients with vascular or nerve invasion was lower (29.7% vs. 62.2% for vascular invasion (P < 0.003) and 29.6% vs. 57.7% for peri-nervous sheathing (P < 0.003). In 2005, Pagès et al showed that 5-year recurrence-free survival dropped from 32.4% to 12.1% in patients with lymphatic and/or vascular tumor emboli and peri-nervous sheathing in their sample of 959 patients operated on for colon cancer(98). These results were reinforced by studies by Stenrberg et al and Liebig et al. (99).

With regard to the comparison of histological prognostic factors according to laterality, several studies have confirmed that right-sided colon cancer is more frequently accompanied by histological factors of poor prognosis(100). In 2017, the study by Lim et al ,including 414 patients operated on between January 2000 and December 2012, showed that right colon cancer presented more lymphatic, vascular and poorly differentiated emboli(86). More recently, in 2019, a study by Helvaci et al including 1,725 patients (1,436 with left colon cancer and 289 with right colon cancer) concluded that right colon cancer presented more lymphatic and vascular invasion, peri-nerve engulfment (21.7% vs. 16%; p=0.046); mucinous subtype (15.2% vs. 7.3%; p<0.001) and poorly differentiated tumors (13.5% vs. 5.4%; p<0.001), giving it a poor prognosis.(101).

In our study, peri-nervous sheathing, vascular and lymphatic emboli are poor prognostic factors for overall and recurrence-free survival. With regard to laterality, our series showed no significant differences in terms of histological characteristics. However, cancer of the right colon appears to be more frequently accompanied by peri-nervous sheathing, vascular and lymphatic emboli, with no significant difference.

3.2.5. Molecular and genetic factors

The genetic study of colon cancers has identified three main alternative mechanisms of carcinogenesis: chromosomal instability, microsatellite instability and epigenetic instability (102). These mechanisms may act separately or concomitantly in colon cancer neogenesis, resulting in distinct genotypes and phenotypes(103,104). These molecular and chromosomal characteristics appear to differ according to tumor site.

- The first mechanism: microsatellite instability (MSI):

It is characterized by hyper-mutable cancers, due to a dysfunction in the DNA mismatch repair system during replication.

The microsatellite unstable phenotype (MSI) is an important colonic carcinogenic pathway detected in around 15% of operable colon cancers(105). It is an important molecular prognostic marker and appears to predict lack of efficacy of adjuvant chemotherapy with 5-FU alone(106). Several studies have shown that colon tumors with MSI-Hight status have better survival than MSS tumors in the early stages of the disease(107-109).

Right colon tumors are generally diploid with a higher rate of microsatellite instability(110). In 2018, Narayanan et al showed that right colon cancers are more aggressive, with higher levels of microsatellite instability and KRAS mutation, which impairs survival, especially in the advanced stages of the disease.(111).

- The second mechanism: chromosomal instability

It is characterized by a high frequency of DNA copy number alterations with non-mutable tumors. It is the first major mechanism of carcinogenesis in colon cancer. This pathway contributes to approximately 75% of GCC versus 25% of DCC (112).

Mutations in the adenomatous polyposis coli (APC) gene have been observed mainly in the GCC(113). They are responsible for sporadic forms of colon cancer and for one of the major forms of hereditary predisposition to colorectal cancer (familial adenomatous polyposis (FAP)).

Mutation of the p53 tumor suppressor gene is more frequent in GCC than in CCD (45% vs. 34%). (112).

- KRAS gene mutation

Kirsten Ras (KRAS) gene activation may follow APC gene inactivation during tumor progression(8)independent of tumour location (114).

Although KRAS mutation is a predictive factor for resistance to anti EGFR, its impact on prognosis has not been clearly established(115). Some studies have reported a poorer prognosis and survival in the presence of these mutations, notably at chromosome 12 and 13(116) such as that by Cejas et al, which showed a higher rate of pulmonary metastases and shorter disease-free survival(117). Other studies concluded that there was no impact on recurrence-free survival or overall survival(118,119).

Concerning tumor laterality, several studies have shown that right-sided cancer is more associated with KRAS(100,111,120).

- BRAF gene mutation :

The B-Raf proto-oncogene (BRAF) is one of the protein serine/threonine kinases that play an important role in differentiation, proliferation or survival regulation. Activating mutations in the BRAF gene induce stimulation of the RAS/MAPK pathway similar to the activation caused by mutations in the KRAS(121).

BRAF gene mutation is considered a poor prognostic factor in several studies(118,122). It is associated with resistance to anti-EGFR drugs. A study by Souglakos showed that BRAF mutation was associated with a poor prognosis, irrespective of the treatment undertaken(123). It also showed that this mutation is associated with a greater risk of disease progression (p<0.0001) and death (p<0.0001).

A number of studies have shown that BRAF mutation occurs mainly in right-colon tumors(100,124).

- The third mechanism: epigenetic instability

It is characterized by the CpG island methylation phenotype (CIMP).
The frequency of MSI High and CIMP High mutations, which results from the inactivation of numerous genes with suppressive actions on cell proliferation, has shown a progressive increase from the rectum (<2.3%) to the ascending colon (36-40%) (125).

Faced with this multitude of genetic and molecular factors, a group of experts recently identified four subtypes of colorectal cancer based on molecular, biological and clinical factors, and proposed the CMS "Consensus Molecular Subtypes" classification (126) :

- CMS-1 group (MSI, Immune): accounts for 13% of colonic cancers, and is preferentially located in the right colon (70% of right-colon cancers belong to this group). Tumors in this group are characterized by MSI-High tumors, marked immune infiltration, high CIMP (CIMP high= methylating phenotype) and BRAF-mutated tumors. Their prognosis is good in the absence of metastases.

- CMS-2 group (canonical): accounts for 35% of colon cancers, preferentially located in the left colon without microsatellite instability (MSS). They are marked by frequent somatic mutations with overexpression of EGFR and activation of the WNT/MYC pathway. Their prognosis is intermediate.

- CMS-3 (metabolic) group: accounts for 11% of colon cancers and is homogeneously distributed between the right and left colon. They are characterized by frequent KRAS mutations, few somatic mutations and no MSS microsatellite instability in 90% of cases. Their prognosis is intermediate.

- CMS-4 (Mesenchymal) group: accounts for 20% of colonic cancers, with a preference for the left colon. These tumors are characterized by numerous somatic alterations (SCNA high), frequent activation of TGFs and angiogenesis, and often MSI tumors. Their prognosis is poor in metastatic situations.

CONCLUSION

Colorectal cancer is a major public health problem. Its frequency is constantly increasing. The distinction between cancer of the colon and rectum has been well established in favor of colorectal cancer in terms of prognosis. However, the difference between left and right colon cancer remains a hotly debated issue.

With this in mind, we conducted our study, the main objective of which was to assess the impact of right or left tumor location on overall survival and recurrence-free survival. We also assessed the epidemiological, clinical and histological profile of each tumour site.

Our study is retrospective mono-centric descriptive and comparative from January 1, 2013 to December 31, 2017, over a period of 5 years, covering patients operated on for colonic cancer, in the general surgery department of the Habib Bourguiba University Hospital in Sfax. We included all patients who had undergone curative resection, emergency or cold, for colonic adenocarcinoma with histological confirmation by anatomopathological examination of the surgical specimen. Tumors of the ileo-caecal valve and recto-sigmoid hinge, synchronous right and left double tumor localization and tumors deemed unresectable were not included to minimize the risk of selection bias and confounding.

Our population comprised 105 individuals, of whom 27 (26%) had right colon cancer (RCC) and 78 (74%) had left colon cancer (LCC). The mean age was 64.7 years, with a sex ratio of 0.98.

As regards the circumstances in which the disease was discovered, no cases were diagnosed during screening. The tumor was complicated in 51 patients (13 CCD and 38 CCG).

The laparoscopic approach was used for 33.3% of scheduled procedures (5 CCD and 13 CCG).

Postoperative follow-up was straightforward in 55.2% of cases, with a morbidity rate of 44.8% and a mortality rate of 0%. The mean post-operative length of stay was 6.68 days (5.12 days CRC and 7.23 days GCC).

All cases were invasive adenocarcinomas, with tumors graded T3 or higher accounting for 90% of cases, and N+ in 57% of cases.

In response to our objectives, our sample showed no significant differences in terms of overall and recurrence-free survival.

Our analytical study concluded that the common poor prognostic factors for overall survival were: age over 70, arterial hypertension, ASA score greater than or equal to II, intraoperative finding of a perforated tumour or a tumour of significant size (greater than 3 cm for the right colon or greater than 5 cm for the left colon), and pathological examination showing peri-nervous sheathing, vascular and/or lymphatic emboli. In addition to the common factors already mentioned, our sample showed specific factors according to laterality: on the one hand, the intraoperative finding of peritonitis or locoregional invasion, and a pathological examination showing a T4 tumour, are factors with a poor prognosis in patients with right-sided colon cancer. On the other hand, the intraoperative finding of liver metastases and the presence of lymph node involvement on pathological examination are considered poor prognostic factors for overall survival in patients with left-sided colon cancer.

With regard to recurrence-free survival, our study concluded that the common poor prognostic factors for patients with right or left colon cancer are: age over 70, intraoperative finding of a perforated or large tumor, and the presence of perineural sheathing or vascular and/or lymphatic emboli on pathological examination. In addition, other statistically significant factors of poor prognosis on recurrence-free survival specific to each location were identified. Factors specific to the right side were the intraoperative finding of peritonitis or the presence of a tumour greater than T3 on pathological examination. For the left side, the specific factors are: ASA score greater than II, intraoperative finding of hepatic metastases, surgery in an emergency context and the presence of lymph node invasion on pathological examination.

Comparison of the epidemiological, clinical and histological profile of each tumor site revealed several statistically significant factors. Diabetes and the presence of an abdominal mass on clinical examination were more frequent in the right colon cancer group (p=0.045 and p=0.04 respectively). Left colon tumors were more frequently associated with synchronous liver metastases (p=0.045) and longer operative times than right colon tumors (p=0.042).

The main limitation of our study is its retrospective nature, which induces a risk of several biases. In addition, the limited number of patients, especially in the right colon cancer group, could influence the results of our study by reducing its power. Furthermore, the molecular characteristics of the tumor, such as MSS/MSI phenotype, BRAF, KRAS and CIMP mutations, which currently represent important prognostic elements in the literature, were not evaluated in our study.

Consequently, we feel that a high-level validation of our results is mandatory in the context of a prospective multicenter study that investigates the different characteristics according to tumor laterality on a larger sample, with the same operative protocol, while of course studying the molecular and genetic characteristics of the tumor. The aim is to refine and target the management of colonic tumors according to their location and characteristics, with a view to personalized (à la carte) therapy for each patient.

At the end of our work, we must stress the importance of colon cancer screening and the development of a well-coded, multidimensional protocol for disseminating information and providing the necessary equipment. Screening is the key to early diagnosis of this cancer, and thus to a definite improvement in prognosis.

REFERENCES

1. Ferlay, J., Ervik, M., Lam, F., Colombet, M., Mery, L., & Piñeros, M.. World Cancer Observatory: "Cancer Today". Lyon: International Agency for Research on Cancer, 2020:1.

2. Rejaibi S, Mahfoudh Mchirgui R, Ben Mansour N, Barbouch F, Kaddour N, Mrabet A, et al. Colorectal cancer mass screening, Tunisia 2019. Evaluation of a pilot program in the Tunis region (Tunisia, 2019). Tunis Med. 1 Jan 2021;99(1):158-67.

3. Xu M, Wu J, Wang C, Huo J, Lü L. [Clinicopathological differences in laterally spreading tumors between rectum and colon]. Zhong Nan Da Xue Xue Bao Yi Xue Ban. 28 Feb 2018;43(2):192-7.

4. Gh L, G M, A A, D B, Ho AH, Sk C. Is right-sided colon cancer different to left-sided colorectal cancer? . European journal of surgical oncology: the journal of the European Society of Surgical Oncology and the British Association of Surgical Oncology. 2015

5. Nawa T, Kato J, Kawamoto H, Okada H, Yamamoto H, Kohno H, et al. Differences between right- and left-sided colon cancer in patient characteristics, cancer morphology and histology. J Gastroenterol Hepatol. March 2008;23(3):418-23.

6. Benedix F, Kube R, Meyer F, Schmidt U, Gastinger I, Lippert H; Colon/Rectum Carcinomas (Primary Tumor) Study Group. Comparison of 17,641 patients with right- and left-sided colon cancer: differences in epidemiology, perioperative course, histology, and survival. Dis Colon Rectum. 2010 Jan;53(1):57-64.

7. Blackburn SA, Parks RM, Cheung KL. Fulvestrant for the treatment of advanced breast cancer. Expert Rev Anticancer Ther. 2018 Jul;18(7):619-628

8. Baran B, Mert Ozupek N, Yerli Tetik N, Acar E, Bekcioglu O, Baskin Y. Difference Between Left-Sided and Right-Sided Colorectal Cancer: A Focused Review of Literature. Gastroenterology Res. 2018 Aug;11(4):264-273.

9. ROUVIÈRE, Henri, DELMAS, André, and DELMAS, Vincent. Système nerveux central, voies et centers nerveux. Masson, 2002.

10. Zinebi A, Eddou H, Moudden KM, Elbaaj M. Etiological profile of anemia in a department of internal medicine [Profil étiologique des anémies dans un service de médecine interne]. Pan Afr Med J. 2017 Jan 4;26:10.

11. Rink AD, Kienle P, Aigner F, Ulrich A. How to reduce anastomotic leakage in colorectal surgery-report from German expert meeting. Langenbecks Arch Surg. 2020 Mar;405(2):223-232.

12. Sciuto A, Merola G, De Palma GD, Sodo M, Pirozzi F, Bracale UM, Bracale U. Predictive factors for anastomotic leakage after laparoscopic colorectal surgery. World J Gastroenterol. 2018 Jun 7;24(21):2247-2260.

13. Fahy BN. Follow-up after curative resection of colorectal cancer. Ann Surg Oncol. 2014 Mar;21(3):738-46.

14. Benedix F, Meyer F, Kube R, Gastinger I, Lippert H. Karzinome des rechten und linken Kolons - verschiedene Tumorentitäten? [Right- and left-sided colonic cancer - different tumour entities]. Zentralbl Chir. 2010 Aug;135(4):312-7. German.

15. Meguid RA, Slidell MB, Wolfgang CL, Chang DC, Ahuja N. Is There a Difference in Survival Between Right-Versus Left-Sided Colon Cancers? Ann Surg Oncol. Sept 2008;15(9):2388-94.

16. Petrelli F, Tomasello G, Borgonovo K, Ghidini M, Turati L, Dallera P, et al. Prognostic Survival Associated With Left-Sided vs Right-Sided Colon Cancer: A Systematic Review and Meta-analysis. JAMA Oncol. 1 Feb 2017;3(2):211-9.

17. Warschkow R, Sulz MC, Marti L, Tarantino I, Schmied BM, Cerny T, Güller U. Better survival in right-sided versus left-sided stage I - III colon cancer patients. BMC Cancer. 2016 Jul 28;16:554.

18. Yang KM, Park IJ, Lee JL, Yoon YS, Kim CW, Lim SB, et al. Does the Different Locations of Colon Cancer Affect the Oncologic Outcome? A Propensity-Score Matched Analysis. Ann Coloproctol. Feb 2019;35(1):15-23.

19. Wang CB, Shahjehan F, Merchea A, Li Z, Bekaii-Saab TS, Grothey A, Colibaseanu DT, Kasi PM. Impact of Tumor Location and Variables Associated With Overall Survival in Patients With Colorectal Cancer: A Mayo Clinic Colon and Rectal Cancer Registry Study. Front Oncol. 2019 Feb 19;9:76.

20. Metin Keskin, Emre Sivrikoz, Gülçin Yeğen, Adem Bayraktar, Cemil Burak Kulle, Dursun Buğra, Mehmet Türker Bulut, Emre Balık.Right vs Left Colon Cancers Have Comparable Survival: a Decade's Experience. Indian Journal of Surgery, 2020; 82(2):134-141.

21. Elferink MA, Visser O, Wiggers T, Otter R, Tollenaar RA, Langendijk JA, Siesling S. Prognostic factors for locoregional

recurrences in colon cancer. Ann Surg Oncol. 2012 Jul;19(7):2203-11.

22. Cienfuegos JA, Baixauli J, Arredondo J, Pastor C, Martínez Ortega P, Zozaya G, Martí-Cruchaga P, Hernández Lizoáin JL. Clinico-pathological and oncological differences between right and left-sided colon cancer (stages I-III): analysis of 950 cases. Rev Esp Enferm Dig. 2018 Mar;110(3):138-144.

23. Moritani K, Hasegawa H, Okabayashi K, Ishii Y, Endo T, Kitagawa Y. Difference in the recurrence rate between right- and left-sided colon cancer: a 17-year experience at a single institution. Surg Today. 2014 Sep;44(9):1685-91.

24. Park JH, Kim MJ, Park SC, Kim MJ, Hong CW, Sohn DK, Han KS, Oh JH. Difference in Time to Locoregional Recurrence Between Patients With Right-Sided and Left-Sided Colon Cancers. Dis Colon Rectum. 2015 Sep;58(9):831-7.

25. Qin Q, Yang L, Sun YK, Ying JM, Song Y, Zhang W, Wang JW, Zhou AP. Comparison of 627 patients with right- and left-sided colon cancer in China: Differences in clinicopathology, recurrence, and survival. Chronic Dis Transl Med. 2017 Mar 13;3(1):51-59.

26. Lee JM, Han YD, Cho MS, Hur H, Min BS, Lee KY, Kim NK. Impact of tumor sidedness on survival and recurrence patterns in colon cancer patients. Ann Surg Treat Res. 2019 Jun;96(6):296-304.

27. Thillainadesan J, Yumol MF, Suen M, Hilmer S, Naganathan V. Enhanced Recovery After Surgery in Older Adults Undergoing Colorectal Surgery: A Systematic Review and Meta-analysis of

Randomized Controlled Trials. Dis Colon Rectum. 2021 Aug 1;64(8):1020-1028.

28. Fernandes R, Shaikh I, Doughan S. Outcomes of elective laparoscopic colorectal operations in octogenarians at a district general hospital in South East England. World J Gastrointest Surg. 2013 Jan 27;5(1):9-11.

29. Newland RC, Dent OF, Lyttle MN, Chapuis PH, Bokey EL. Pathologic determinants of survival associated with colorectal cancer with lymph node metastases. A multivariate analysis of 579 patients. Cancer. 1994 Apr 15;73(8):2076-82.

30. Chapuis PH, Dent OF, Fisher R, Newland RC, Pheils MT, Smyth E, Colquhoun K. A multivariate analysis of clinical and pathological variables in prognosis after resection of large bowel cancer. Br J Surg. 1985 Sep;72(9):698-702.

31. Park HC, Shin A, Kim BW, Jung KW, Won YJ, Oh JH, et al. Data on the Characteristics and the Survival of Korean Patients With Colorectal Cancer From the Korea Central Cancer Registry. Ann Coloproctol. August 2013;29(4):144-9.

32. Nakagawa-Senda H, Hori M, Matsuda T, Ito H. Prognostic impact of tumor location in colon cancer: the Monitoring of Cancer Incidence in Japan (MCIJ) project. BMC Cancer. May 2019;19(1):431.

33. Turner MC, Becerra D, Sun Z, Watson J, Leung K, Migaly J, et al. The side of the primary tumor affects overall survival in colon adenocarcinoma: an analysis of the national cancer database. Tech Coloproctol. June 2019;23(6):537-44.

34. Tapia Rico G, Price T, Tebbutt N, Hardingham J, Lee C, Buizen L, et al. Right or Left Primary Site of Colorectal Cancer: Outcomes From the Molecular Analysis of the AGITG MAX Trial. Clin Colorectal Cancer. 2019;18(2):141-8.

35. Biondo S, Gálvez A, Ramírez E, Frago R, Kreisler E. Emergency surgery for obstructing and perforated colon cancer: patterns of recurrence and prognostic factors. Tech Coloproctol. 2019 Dec;23(12):1141-1161.

36. Radespiel-Tröger M, Hohenberger W, Reingruber B. Improved prediction of recurrence after curative resection of colon carcinoma using tree-based risk stratification. Cancer. 2004 Mar 1;100(5):958-67.

37. Jess P, Hansen IO, Gamborg M, Jess T; Danish Colorectal Cancer Group. A nationwide Danish cohort study challenging the categorisation into right-sided and left-sided colon cancer. BMJ Open. 2013 May 28;3(5):e002608.

38. Seydaoğlu G, Özer B, Arpacı N, Parsak CK, Eray IC. Trends in colorectal cancer by subsite, age, and gender over a 15-year period in Adana, Turkey: 1993-2008. Turk J Gastroenterol. 2013;24(6):521-31.

39. NEHAOUA, Amine. Obesity, psychosocial representations and stigmatization, pathophysiological consequences: diagnosis and management through physical and sports activities. 2021.

40. Sinicrope FA, Foster NR, Yothers G, Benson A, Seitz JF, Labianca R, Goldberg RM, Degramont A, O'Connell MJ, Sargent DJ; Adjuvant Colon Cancer Endpoints (ACCENT) Group. Body mass index at

diagnosis and survival among colon cancer patients enrolled in clinical trials of adjuvant chemotherapy. Cancer. 2013 Apr 15;119(8):1528-36.

41. Brulé SY, Jonker DJ, Karapetis CS, O'Callaghan CJ, Moore MJ, Wong R, et al. Location of colon cancer (right-sided versus left-sided) as a prognostic factor and a predictor of benefit from cetuximab in NCIC CO.17. Eur J Cancer. jul 2015;51(11):1405-14.

42. Weijenberg MP, Aardening PW, de Kok TM, de Goeij AF, van den Brandt PA. Cigarette smoking and KRAS oncogene mutations in sporadic colorectal cancer: results from the Netherlands Cohort Study. Mutat Res. 2008 Mar 29;652(1):54-64.

43. Terry P, Ekbom A, Lichtenstein P, Feychting M, Wolk A. Long-term tobacco smoking and colorectal cancer in a prospective cohort study. Int J Cancer. 2001 Feb 15;91(4):585-7.

44. Wu AH, Henderson BE. Alcohol and tobacco use: risk factors for colorectal adenoma and carcinoma? J Natl Cancer Inst. 1995 Feb 15;87(4):239-40.

45. Yancik R, Wesley MN, Ries LA, Havlik RJ, Long S, Edwards BK, Yates JW. Comorbidity and age as predictors of risk for early mortality of male and female colon carcinoma patients: a population-based study. Cancer. 1998 Jun 1;82(11):2123-34.

46. Nitsche U, Späth C, Müller TC, Maak M, Janssen KP, Wilhelm D, Kleeff J, Bader FG. Colorectal cancer surgery remains effective with rising patient age. Int J Colorectal Dis. 2014 Aug;29(8):971-9.

47. Park JH, Kim DH, Kim BR, Kim YW. The American Society of Anesthesiologists score influences on postoperative complications and total hospital charges after laparoscopic colorectal cancer surgery. Medicine (Baltimore). 2018 May;97(18):e0653.

48. Sarikaya H, Benhidjeb T, Iosivan SI, Kolokotronis T, Förster C, Eckert S, Wilkens L, Nasser A, Rehberg S, Krüger M, Schulte Am Esch J. Impact of ASA-score, age and learning curve on early outcome in the initiation phase of an oncological robotic colorectal program. Sci Rep. 2020 Sep 15;10(1):15136.

49. Stein KB, Snyder CF, Barone BB, Yeh HC, Peairs KS, Derr RL, Wolff AC, Brancati FL. Colorectal cancer outcomes, recurrence, and complications in persons with and without diabetes mellitus: a systematic review and meta-analysis. Dig Dis Sci. 2010 Jul;55(7):1839-51.

50. Wang C, Wainberg ZA, Raldow A, Lee P. Differences in Cancer-Specific Mortality of Right- Versus Left-Sided Colon Adenocarcinoma: A Surveillance, Epidemiology, and End Results Database Analysis. JCO Clin Cancer Inform. 2017;1:1-9.

51. Burton S, Norman AR, Brown G, Abulafi AM, Swift RI. Predictive poor prognostic factors in colonic carcinoma. Surg Oncol. 2006 Aug;15(2):71-8.

52. Cheynel N, Cortet M, Lepage C, Ortega-Debalon P, Faivre J, Bouvier AM. Incidence, patterns of failure, and prognosis of perforated colorectal cancers in a well-defined population. Dis Colon Rectum. 2009 Mar;52(3):406-11.

53. Ho YH, Siu SK, Buttner P, Stevenson A, Lumley J, Stitz R. The effect of obstruction and perforation on colorectal cancer disease-free survival. World J Surg. 2010 May;34(5):1091-101.

54. Yang KM, Jeong MJ, Yoon KH, Jung YT, Kwak JY. Oncologic outcome of colon cancer with perforation and obstruction. BMC Gastroenterol. 2022 May 15;22(1):247.

55. Saha S, Shaik M, Johnston G, Saha SK, Berbiglia L, Hicks M, Gernand J, Grewal S, Arora M, Wiese D. Tumor size predicts long-term survival in colon cancer: an analysis of the National Cancer Data Base. Am J Surg. 2015 Mar;209(3):570-4.

56. Korant, Alpesh MD[1] ; Shaik, Mohammed MD[2] ; Saha, Supriya MD[3] ; Gay, Greer PhD[4] ; Saha, Sukamal MD[1] . Tumor Size Predicts Long-Term Survival in Colon Cancer Patients: Analysis of National Cancer Database (NCDB): Presidential Poster: 550. American Journal of Gastroenterology: 2013October - Volume 108 - Issue - p S162

57. Kornprat P, Pollheimer MJ, Lindtner RA, Schlemmer A, Rehak P, Langner C. Value of tumor size as a prognostic variable in colorectal cancer: a critical reappraisal. Am J Clin Oncol. 2011 Feb;34(1):43-9.

58. Liang Y, Li Q, He D, Chen Y, Li J. Tumor size improves the accuracy of the prognostic prediction of T4a stage colon cancer. Sci Rep. 2021 Aug 11;11(1):16264.

59. Alese OB, Zhou W, Jiang R, Zakka K, Huang Z, Okoli C, Shaib WL, Akce M, Diab M, Wu C, El-Rayes BF. Predictive and Prognostic Effects of Primary Tumor Size on Colorectal Cancer Survival. Front Oncol. 2021 Dec 9;11:728076.

60. Papagiorgis P, Oikonomakis I, Karapanagiotou I, Wexner SD, Nikiteas N. The impact of tumor location on the histopathologic expression of colorectal cancer. J BUON. Sept 2006;11(3):317-21.

61. Nawa T, Kato J, Kawamoto H, Okada H, Yamamoto H, Kohno H, et al. Differences between right- and left-sided colon cancer in patient characteristics, cancer morphology and histology. J Gastroenterol Hepatol. March 2008;23(3):418-23.

62. Holleczek B, Rossi S, Domenic A, Innos K, Minicozzi P, Francisci S, et al. On-going improvement and persistent differences in the survival for patients with colon and rectum cancer across Europe 1999-2007 - Results from the EUROCARE-5 study. Eur J Cancer. oct 2015;51(15):2158-68.

63. Gupta A, Gupta E, Hilsden R, Hawel JD, Elnahas AI, Schlachta CM, Alkhamesi NA. Preoperative malnutrition in patients with colorectal cancer. Can J Surg. 2021 Nov 25;64(6):E621-E629.

64. Nazha B, Moussaly E, Zaarour M, Weerasinghe C, Azab B. Hypoalbuminemia in colorectal cancer prognosis: Nutritional marker or inflammatory surrogate? World J Gastrointest Surg. 2015 Dec 27;7(12):370-7.

65. Almasaudi AS, Dolan RD, Edwards CA, McMillan DC. Hypoalbuminemia Reflects Nutritional Risk, Body Composition and Systemic Inflammation and Is Independently Associated with Survival in Patients with Colorectal Cancer. Cancers (Basel). 2020 Jul 21;12(7):1986.

66. Fujii T, Sutoh T, Morita H, Katoh T, Yajima R, Tsutsumi S, et al. Serum Albumin Is Superior to Prealbumin for Predicting Short-Term

Recurrence in Patients with Operable Colorectal Cancer. Nutrition and Cancer. 1 Nov 2012;64(8):1169-73.

67. Ding PR, An X, Zhang RX, Fang YJ, Li LR, Chen G, Wu XJ, Lu ZH, Lin JZ, Kong LH, Wan DS, Pan ZZ. Elevated preoperative neutrophil to lymphocyte ratio predicts risk of recurrence following curative resection for stage IIA colon cancer. Int J Colorectal Dis. 2010 Dec;25(12):1427-33.

68. Mallappa S, Sinha A, Gupta S, Chadwick SJ. Preoperative neutrophil to lymphocyte ratio >5 is a prognostic factor for recurrent colorectal cancer. Colorectal Dis. 2013 Mar;15(3):323-8.

69. Liao CK, Yu YL, Lin YC, Hsu YJ, Chern YJ, Chiang JM, et al. Prognostic value of the C-reactive protein to albumin ratio in colorectal cancer: an updated systematic review and meta-analysis. World Journal of Surgical Oncology. May 2021;19(1):139.

70. Bai Z, Wang J, Wang T, Li Y, Zhao X, Wu G, Yang Y, Deng W, Zhang Z. Clinicopathologic parameters associated with postoperative complications and risk factors for tumor recurrence and mortality after tumor resection of patients with colorectal cancer. Clin Transl Oncol. 2018 Feb;20(2):176-192.

71. Amri R, Bordeianou LG, Sylla P, Berger DL. Preoperative carcinoembryonic antigen as an outcome predictor in colon cancer. J Surg Oncol. 2013 Jul;108(1):14-8.

72. Kim CG, Ahn JB, Jung M, Beom SH, Heo SJ, Kim JH, Kim YJ, Kim NK, Min BS, Koom WS, Kim H, Roh YH, Ma BG, Shin SJ. Preoperative Serum Carcinoembryonic Antigen Level as a Prognostic Factor for Recurrence and Survival After Curative Resection

Followed by Adjuvant Chemotherapy in Stage III Colon Cancer. Ann Surg Oncol. 2017 Jan;24(1):227-235.

73. Kalantzis I, Nonni A, Pavlakis K, Delicha EM, Miltiadou K, Kosmas C, et al. Clinicopathological differences and correlations between right and left colon cancer. World J Clin Cases. 26 Apr 2020;8(8):1424-43.

74. Keeler BD, Mishra A, Stavrou CL, Beeby S, Simpson JA, Acheson AG. A cohort investigation of anaemia, treatment and the use of allogeneic blood transfusion in colorectal cancer surgery. Ann Med Surg (Lond). march 2016;6:6-11.

75. Dunne JR, Gannon CJ, Osborn TM, Taylor MD, Malone DL, Napolitano LM. Preoperative anemia in colon cancer: assessment of risk factors. Am Surg. June 2002;68(6):582-7.

76. Ueno H, Mochizuki H, Hashiguchi Y, Shimazaki H, Aida S, Hase K, Matsukuma S, Kanai T, Kurihara H, Ozawa K, Yoshimura K, Bekku S. Risk factors for an adverse outcome in early invasive colorectal carcinoma. Gastroenterology. 2004 Aug;127(2):385-94.

77. Shepherd NA, Saraga EP, Love SB, Jass JR. Prognostic factors in colonic cancer. Histopathology. 1989 Jun;14(6):613-20.

78. Quah HM, Chou JF, Gonen M, Shia J, Schrag D, Landmann RG, Guillem JG, Paty PB, Temple LK, Wong WD, Weiser MR. Identification of patients with high-risk stage II colon cancer for adjuvant therapy. Dis Colon Rectum. 2008 May;51(5):503-7.

79. Böckelman C, Engelmann BE, Kaprio T, Hansen TF, Glimelius B. Risk of recurrence in patients with colon cancer stage II and III: a

systematic review and meta-analysis of recent literature. Acta Oncol. 2015 Jan;54(1):5-16.

80. Macari D, Kawak S, Raofi V, Wasvary H, Jaiyesimi I. Recurrence pattern and outcomes in T4 colon cancer: A single institution analysis. Journal of Surgical Oncology. February 2020;121(2):337-41.

81. Liska D, Stocchi L, Karagkounis G, Elagili F, Dietz DW, Kalady MF, Kessler H, Remzi FH, Church J. Incidence, Patterns, and Predictors of Locoregional Recurrence in Colon Cancer. Ann Surg Oncol. 2017 Apr;24(4):1093-1099.

82. Ogino S, Nosho K, Irahara N, Shima K, Baba Y, Kirkner GJ, et al. Negative Lymph Node Count Is Associated With Survival of Colorectal Cancer Patients, Independent of Tumoral Molecular Alterations and Lymphocytic Reaction. Am J Gastroenterol. Feb 2010;105(2):420-33.

83. Chang GJ, Rodriguez-Bigas MA, Skibber JM, Moyer VA. Lymph node evaluation and survival after curative resection of colon cancer: systematic review. J Natl Cancer Inst. 2007 Mar 21;99(6):433-41.

84. Elferink MAG, Siesling S, Visser O, Rutten HJ, van Krieken JHJM, Tollenaar RAEM, Lemmens VEPP. Large variation between hospitals and pathology laboratories in lymph node evaluation in colon cancer and its impact on survival, a nationwide population-based study in the Netherlands. Ann Oncol. 2011 Jan;22(1):110-117.

85. Marzouk O, Schofield J. Review of histopathological and molecular prognostic features in colorectal cancer. Cancers (Basel). 2011 Jun 23;3(2):2767-810.

86. Lim DR, Kuk JK, Kim T, Shin EJ. Comparison of oncological outcomes of right-sided colon cancer versus left-sided colon cancer after curative resection: Which side is better outcome? Medicine (Baltimore). oct 2017;96(42):e8241.

87. Yang CY, Yen MH, Kiu KT, Chen YT, Chang TC. Outcomes of right-sided and left-sided colon cancer after curative resection. Sci Rep. 5 Jul 2022;12(1):11323.

88. Kobayashi H, West NP, Takahashi K, Perrakis A, Weber K, Hohenberger W, Quirke P, Sugihara K. Quality of surgery for stage III colon cancer: comparison between England, Germany, and Japan. Ann Surg Oncol. 2014 Jun;21 Suppl 3:S398-404.

89. Kessler H, Hohenberger W. Extended lymphadenectomy in colon cancer is crucial. World J Surg. 2013 Aug;37(8):1789-98.

90. Compton CC. Colorectal carcinoma: diagnostic, prognostic, and molecular features. Mod Pathol. 2003 Apr;16(4):376-88.

91. Choi PW, Yu CS, Jang SJ, Jung SH, Kim HC, Kim JC. Risk factors for lymph node metastasis in submucosal invasive colorectal cancer. World J Surg. 2008 Sep;32(9):2089-94.

92. Carraro PG, Segala M, Cesana BM, Tiberio G. Obstructing colonic cancer: failure and survival patterns over a ten-year follow-up after one-stage curative surgery. Dis Colon Rectum. 2001 Feb;44(2):243-50.

93. Börger ME, Gosens MJ, Jeuken JW, van Kempen LC, van de Velde CJ, van Krieken JH, Nagtegaal ID. Signet ring cell differentiation in mucinous colorectal carcinoma. J Pathol. 2007 Jul;212(3):278-86.

94. O'Connell JB, Maggard MA, Ko CY. Colon cancer survival rates with the new American Joint Committee on Cancer sixth edition staging. J Natl Cancer Inst. 2004 Oct 6;96(19):1420-5.

95. Law WL, Chu KW. Anterior resection for rectal cancer with mesorectal excision: a prospective evaluation of 622 patients. Ann Surg. 2004 Aug;240(2):260-8.

96. H M, A M, H K, Y N, A I, Y O, et al. Venous invasion and down-regulation of p21(WAF1/CIP1) are associated with metastasis in colorectal carcinomas. Hepatogastroenterology. 1 Sep 2005; 52(65):1421-6.

97. Krasna MJ, Flancbaum L, Cody RP, Shneibaum S, Ben Ari G. Vascular and neural invasion in colorectal carcinoma. Incidence and prognostic significance. Cancer. 1988 Mar 1;61(5):1018-23.

98. Pagès F, Berger A, Camus M, Sanchez-Cabo F, Costes A, Molidor R, Mlecnik B, Kirilovsky A, Nilsson M, Damotte D, Meatchi T, Bruneval P, Cugnenc PH, Trajanoski Z, Fridman WH, Galon J. Effector memory T cells, early metastasis, and survival in colorectal cancer. N Engl J Med. 2005 Dec 22;353(25):2654-66.

99. Liebig C, Ayala G, Wilks J, Verstovsek G, Liu H, Agarwal N, Berger DH, Albo D. Perineural invasion is an independent predictor of outcome in colorectal cancer. J Clin Oncol. 2009 Nov 1;27(31):5131-7.

100. Hsu YL, Lin CC, Jiang JK, Lin HH, Lan YT, Wang HS, et al. Clinicopathological and molecular differences in colorectal cancer according to location. Int J Biol Markers. March 1, 2019;34(1):47-53.

101. Kaan Helvaci, Emrah Eraslan, Fatih Yildiz, Gulnihal Tufan, Umut Demirci, Omur Berna Oksuzoglu, Ulku Yalcintas Arslan. JBUON. 2019; 24(5): 1845-1851

102. Boland CR, Goel A. Microsatellite instability in colorectal cancer. Gastroenterology. June 2010;138(6):2073-2087.

103. Hinoue T, Weisenberger DJ, Lange CPE, Shen H, Byun HM, Van Den Berg D, et al. Genome-scale analysis of aberrant DNA methylation in colorectal cancer. Genome Res. Feb 2012;22(2):271-82.

104. Kudryavtseva AV, Lipatova AV, Zaretsky AR, Moskalev AA, Fedorova MS, Rasskazova AS, et al. Important molecular genetic markers of colorectal cancer. Oncotarget. August 16, 2016;7(33):53959-83.

105. Sinicrope FA, Sargent DJ. Clinical implications of microsatellite instability in sporadic colon cancers. Curr Opin Oncol. Jul 2009;21(4):369-73.

106. Predictive and prognostic value of the MSI phenotype in non-metastatic colon cancer: who and how to treat? Cancer Bulletin. Feb 1, 2019; 106(2):129-36.

107. Lawes DA, SenGupta S, Boulos PB. The clinical importance and prognostic implications of microsatellite instability in sporadic cancer. Eur J Surg Oncol. 2003 Apr;29(3):201-12.

108. Elsaleh H, Iacopetta B. Microsatellite instability is a predictive marker for survival benefit from adjuvant chemotherapy in a

population-based series of stage III colorectal carcinoma. Clin Colorectal Cancer. 2001 Aug;1(2):104-9.

109. Ribic CM, Sargent DJ, Moore MJ, Thibodeau SN, French AJ, Goldberg RM, Hamilton SR, Laurent-Puig P, Gryfe R, Shepherd LE, Tu D, Redston M, Gallinger S. Tumor microsatellite-instability status as a predictor of benefit from fluorouracil-based adjuvant chemotherapy for colon cancer. N Engl J Med. 2003 Jul 17;349(3):247-57.

110. Sugai T, Habano W, Jiao YF, Tsukahara M, Takeda Y, Otsuka K, et al. Analysis of Molecular Alterations in Left- and Right-Sided Colorectal Carcinomas Reveals Distinct Pathways of Carcinogenesis. J Mol Diagn. May 2006;8(2):193-201.

111. Narayanan S, Gabriel E, Attwood K, Boland P, Nurkin S. Association of Clinicopathologic and Molecular Markers on Stage-specific Survival of Right Versus Left Colon Cancer. Clin Colorectal Cancer. 2018;17(4):671-8.

112. Shen H, Yang J, Huang Q, Jiang MJ, Tan YN, Fu JF, et al. Different treatment strategies and molecular features between right-sided and left-sided colon cancers. World Journal of Gastroenterology. 2015 June 7;21(21):6470-8

113. Zhang L, Shay JW. Multiple Roles of APC and its Therapeutic Implications in Colorectal Cancer. J Natl Cancer Inst. 01 2017;109(8).

114. Arnold D, Lueza B, Douillard JY, Peeters M, Lenz HJ, Venook A, et al. Prognostic and predictive value of primary tumour side in patients with RAS wild-type metastatic colorectal cancer treated with

chemotherapy and EGFR directed antibodies in six randomized trials. Ann Oncol. August 1, 2017;28(8):1713-29.

115. Di Fiore F, Michel P. Prognostic role of KRAS mutation in colorectal cancer. Bull Cancer. 2009 Dec;96 Suppl:S23-30.

116. Andreyev HJ, Norman AR, Cunningham D, Oates J, Dix BR, Iacopetta BJ, Young J, Walsh T, Ward R, Hawkins N, Beranek M, Jandik P, Benamouzig R, Jullian E, Laurent-Puig P, Olschwang S, Muller O, Hoffmann I, Rabes HM, Zietz C, Troungos C, Valavanis C, Yuen ST, Ho JW, Croke CT, O'Donoghue DP, Giaretti W, Rapallo A, Russo A, Bazan V, Tanaka M, Omura K, Azuma T, Ohkusa T, Fujimori T, Ono Y, Pauly M, Faber C, Glaesener R, de Goeij AF, Arends JW, Andersen SN, Lövig T, Breivik J, Gaudernack G, Clausen OP, De Angelis PD, Meling GI, Rognum TO, Smith R, Goh HS, Font A, Rosell R, Sun XF, Zhang H, Benhattar J, Losi L, Lee JQ, Wang ST, Clarke PA, Bell S, Quirke P, Bubb VJ, Piris J, Cruickshank NR, Morton D, Fox JC, Al-Mulla F, Lees N, Hall CN, Snary D, Wilkinson K, Dillon D, Costa J, Pricolo VE, Finkelstein SD, Thebo JS, Senagore AJ, Halter SA, Wadler S, Malik S, Krtolica K, Urosevic N. Kirsten ras mutations in patients with colorectal cancer: the 'RASCAL II' study. Br J Cancer. 2001 Sep 1;85(5):692-6.

117 Cejas P, López-Gómez M, Aguayo C, Madero R, Carpeño J de C, Belda-Iniesta C, et al. KRAS Mutations in Primary Colorectal Cancer Tumors and Related Metastases: A Potential Role in Prediction of Lung Metastasis. PLOS ONE. Dec 2009;4(12):e8199.

118. Roth AD, Tejpar S, Delorenzi M, Yan P, Fiocca R, Klingbiel D, Dietrich D, Biesmans B, Bodoky G, Barone C, Aranda E, Nordlinger B, Cisar L, Labianca R, Cunningham D, Van Cutsem E, Bosman F.

Prognostic role of KRAS and BRAF in stage II and III resected colon cancer: results of the translational study on the PETACC-3, EORTC 40993, SAKK 60-00 trial. J Clin Oncol. 2010 Jan 20;28(3):466-74.

119. Ogino S, Meyerhardt JA, Irahara N, Niedzwiecki D, Hollis D, Saltz LB, Mayer RJ, Schaefer P, Whittom R, Hantel A, Benson AB 3rd, Goldberg RM, Bertagnolli MM, Fuchs CS; Cancer and Leukemia Group B; North Central Cancer Treatment Group; Canadian Cancer Society Research Institute; Southwest Oncology Group. KRAS mutation in stage III colon cancer and clinical outcome following intergroup trial CALGB 89803. Clin Cancer Res. 2009 Dec 1;15(23):7322-9.

120. Fric P, Sovová V, Sloncová E, Lojda Z, Jirásek A, Cermák J. Different expression of some molecular markers in sporadic cancer of the left and right colon. Eur J Cancer Prev. 2000 Aug;9(4):265-8.

121. Galmiche A, Ezzoukhry Z. Regulation of cell survival by RAF family kinases. Med Sci (Paris). August 1, 2010; 26(8-9):729-33.

122. Fariña-Sarasqueta A, van Lijnschoten G, Moerland E, Creemers GJ, Lemmens VEPP, Rutten HJT, van den Brule AJC. The BRAF V600E mutation is an independent prognostic factor for survival in stage II and stage III colon cancer patients. Ann Oncol. 2010 Dec;21(12):2396-2402.

123. André T, Meyerhardt J, Iveson T, Sobrero A, Yoshino T, Souglakos I, Grothey A, Niedzwiecki D, Saunders M, Labianca R, Yamanaka T, Boukovinas I, Vernerey D, Meyers J, Harkin A, Torri V, Oki E, Georgoulias V, Taieb J, Shields A, Shi Q. Effect of duration of adjuvant chemotherapy for patients with stage III colon cancer (IDEA

collaboration): final results from a prospective, pooled analysis of six randomised, phase 3 trials. Lancet Oncol. 2020 Dec;21(12):1620-1629.

124. Missiaglia E, Jacobs B, D'Ario G, Di Narzo AF, Soneson C, Budinska E, et al. Distal and proximal colon cancers differ in terms of molecular, pathological, and clinical features. Ann Oncol. oct 2014;25(10):1995-2001.

125. Yamauchi M, Morikawa T, Kuchiba A, Imamura Y, Qian ZR, Nishihara R, Liao X, Waldron L, Hoshida Y, Huttenhower C, Chan AT, Giovannucci E, Fuchs C, Ogino S. Assessment of colorectal cancer molecular features along bowel subsites challenges the conception of distinct dichotomy of proximal versus distal colorectum. Gut. 2012 Jun;61(6):847-54.

126. Guinney J, Dienstmann R, Wang X, de Reyniès A, Schlicker A, Soneson C, et al. The consensus molecular subtypes of colorectal cancer. Nat Med. nov 2015;21(11):1350-6.

APPENDICES

Appendix 1: SCORE ASA

Classes	Description
I	Healthy patient in apparent good health
II	Patients with moderate systemic abnormalities
III	Patients with severe systemic abnormalities
IV	Patients with severe, life-threatening systemic abnormalities
V	Moribund patient unlikely to survive without intervention
IV	Brain-dead patient whose organs are removed for transplantation

Appendix2: TNM classification (8th edition, 2017)

Tis: carcinoma in situ, intramucosal tumor invading the lamina propria (chorion) without extension through the muscularis mucosa to the submucosa.

T1: tumor invading the submucosa

T2: tumor invading the muscularis propria

T3: tumor invading the subserosa or non-peritoneal pericolic and perirectal tissues

T4: tumor directly invading other organs or structures and/or perforating the visceral peritoneum

T4a: tumor perforating the visceral peritoneum

T4b: tumor directly invading other nearby organs or structures

Nx: insufficient information to classify regional adenopathies

N0: no regional lymph node metastasis

N1: metastasis in 1 to 3 regional lymph nodes***.

N1a: metastasis in 1 regional lymph node

N1b: metastases in 2-3 regional lymph nodes

N1c: "satellite" tumour nodule(s) (or deposits) in the subserosa, or in non-peritonealpericolic or perirectal tissues, without regional metastatic lymph node.

N2: metastases $\geq$ 4 regional lymph nodes

N2a: metastases in 4-6 regional lymph nodes

N2b: metastases in $\geq$ 7 regional lymph nodes

M0: no distant metastases

M1: Remote metastasis(es)

M1a: metastasis(es) localized to a single organ (liver, lung, ovary, non-regional lymph node(s)) without peritoneal metastasis

M1b: multi-organ metastases without peritoneal metastases

M1c: peritoneal metastasis(es) with or without metastasis to other organs

Classification by stage

Stage 0	pTis N0 M0
Stage I	pT1-2 N0 M0
Stage IIA	pT3 N0 M0
Stage IIB	pT4a N0 M0
Stage IIC	pT4b N0 M0
Stage IIIA	pT1-T2 N1/N1c M0 and pT1 N2a M0
Stage IIIB	pT3-T4a N1N1c M0, pT2-T3 N2a M0, pT1-T2 N2b M0
Stage IIIC	pT4a N2a M0; p T3-T4a N2b M0; pT4b N1-N2 M0
Stage IVA	all T, all N, M1a
Stage IVB	all T, all N, M1b
IVC stage	all T, all N, M1c

SUMMARY

PROBLEMATIC :

Colon cancer is a public health problem. The differentiation between right and left colon cancer is a topical issue. Indeed, a better understanding of clinico-pathological elements and the distinction of prognostic factors according to tumor location and characteristics could target therapeutic management, thus improving prognosis.

PURPOSE OF WORK :

The primary objective of our study is to evaluate the impact of right or left location of primary colon adenocarcinoma on prognosis (overall survival and recurrence-free survival) in patients after curative surgery. The secondary objective is to evaluate the epidemiological, clinical and histological profile of each tumor site.

MATERIALS AND METHODS :

This is a mono-centric descriptive and comparative retrospective study running from January 1, 2013 to December 31, 2017, i.e. a duration of 5 years, involving patients operated on for colonic cancer, in the Habib Bourguiba general surgery department in Sfax.

RESULTS :

Our population comprised 105 individuals, including 27 (26%) with right-colon tumors and 78 (74%) with left-colon tumors. T3-T4 and N+ tumors accounted for 90% and 60% respectively of our total sample. Comparison of the two groups (right and left colon) showed no significant differences in terms of overall survival and recurrence-free survival.

Our analytical study revealed common poor prognostic factors for both groups in terms of overall survival and recurrence-free survival, notably advanced tumour stage, tumour perforation and the presence of peri-nervous sheathing, vascular and lymphatic emboli on pathological examination. Our sample also showed specific factors according to laterality, notably the presence of peritonitis and locoregional invasion for the right colon, and the presence of lymph node invasion and liver metastases for the left colon.

A comparative study of the epidemiological, clinical and histological profile showed statistically significant differences between right-sided and left-sided colon cancer. On the one hand, the presence of diabetes and the palpation of an abdominal mass on clinical examination are more frequent on the right side. On the other hand, the presence of synchronous liver metastases is more frequent on the left side.

CONCLUSION:

Our study suggests the presence of differences in prognosis, epidemiological, clinical and histological profile according to tumor laterality. High-level validation of our results is essential in the context of a prospective multicenter study. At the end of our work, we must insist on the importance of screening, which is an essential element in the early diagnosis of this cancer, enabling a definite improvement in prognosis.

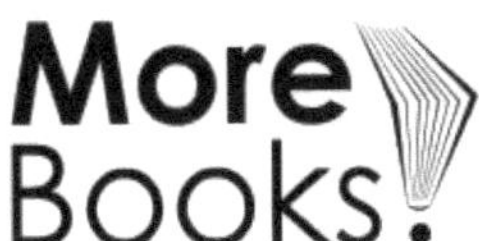

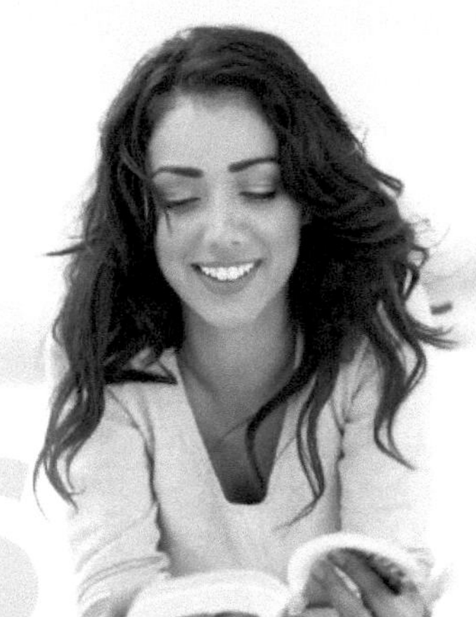

I want morebooks!

Buy your books fast and straightforward online - at one of world's fastest growing online book stores! Environmentally sound due to Print-on-Demand technologies.

Buy your books online at
www.morebooks.shop

Kaufen Sie Ihre Bücher schnell und unkompliziert online – auf einer der am schnellsten wachsenden Buchhandelsplattformen weltweit! Dank Print-On-Demand umwelt- und ressourcenschonend produzi ert.

Bücher schneller online kaufen
www.morebooks.shop

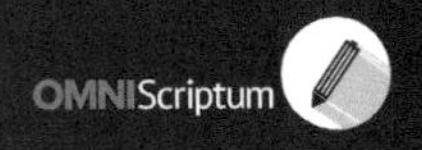

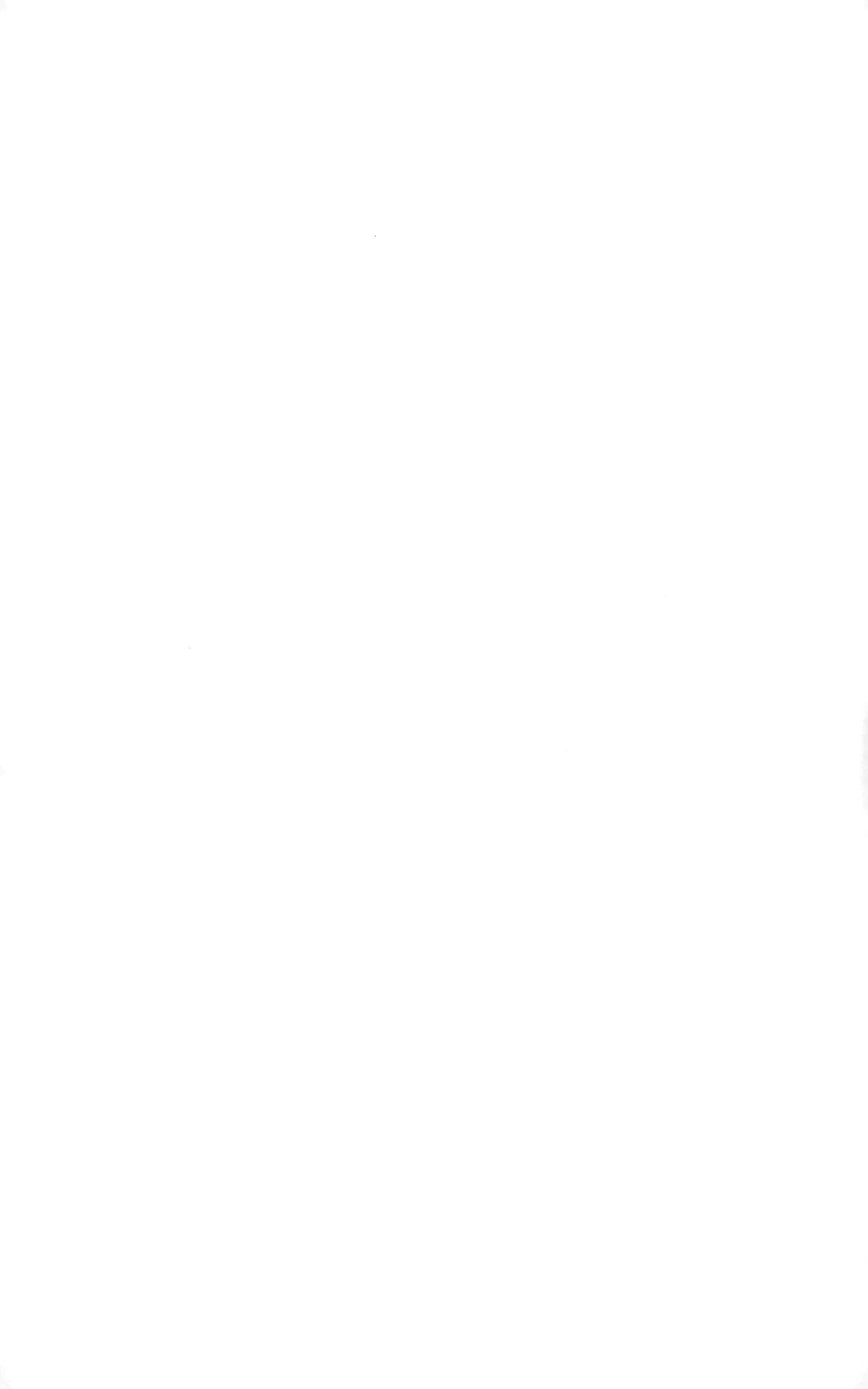

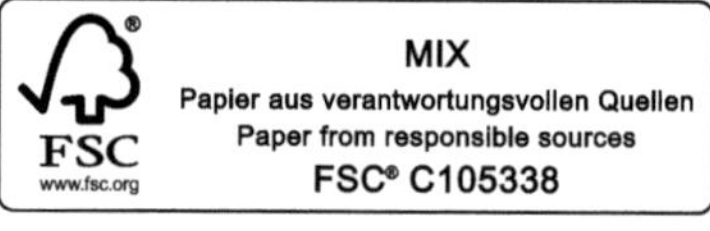

Printed by Books on Demand GmbH, Norderstedt / Germany